WHAT PEOPLE ▲
ABOUT RITA K.

"I attended a Women's Retreat and Rita spoke to us on Simple Self Care which included stretching exercises. I was skeptical that such easy actions would make a difference. I started the lower back stretch and stretch while brushing my teeth. I am amazed at how much better I feel now! I feel stronger and more toned and have more stamina. These simple stretches have led me to more stretching and exercising. Thank you Rita for helping me move more comfortably."

—Beth Brunner:
Neonatal Nurse Practitioner at Carolinas Medical Center Pineville

"My self-care has become an important daily part of my life because of Rita's simple tips provided in our Woman's Advantage Forums for the past year! With Rita as our hosting business for our Forums, she gives a monthly tip to the members that is simple and easy to apply! The results that they see start right away and they see how it impacts their business success, too. Who would think that pausing to breathe would help you to focus with less stress and make more money, too! I highly recommend Rita Garnto and her workshops as an essential part of your personal and business success!"

—Lori Dvorak,
InVision 4, Inc. Vision Strategy Coaching & Training,
The Woman's Advantage Forum, Charlotte Chair

"Rita broadened my awareness of ways I already do self-care, and helped me to recognize the importance of those. She also encouraged me to find new ways to reduce stress and take care of my mental, emotional, physical, and spiritual health each day. Her genuinely compassionate and down-to-earth approach is refreshing!

"Rita has helped me to realize that self-care is not complicated but is quite simple, in all of the small, run-of-the-mill ways we pay attention to our physical, mental, emotional, and spiritual well-being. Her workshops are refreshing and life-giving!"

—Marianne Romanat,
Lead Pastor, Light of Christ United Methodist Church
www.locumc.org

"I can't tell you how much the class you gave on setting your goals and making myself part of my life. Because of you, I could see I need to move in a slower direction on how to be true to myself. One thing that I realized was that when I try to make good choices to move ahead in my life, I try to do everything at once. Your Advice was to take on One Challenge at a Time. Big Lesson for me and your follow-up email that wanted to know how I was doing, made me feel happy that "Someone like YOU Cares! Angels blessing to You, Rita!"

—Selinda B.

"I love working with Rita - who helped me to understand that I don't have to start out with a 90 minute a day cardio/exercise running marathon. She said . . . just a few steps more . . . She understands that simple and easy gets things done. Now I park a little further from the entrance and take a few more steps everywhere I go . . . . Thank you Rita for your encouragement and showing us that busy women can take care of themselves simply and with a smile!!"

—Wendy Cassera, Taxpectations

"The 'Making You a Priority' workshop helped remind me to take time to care for myself. Rita is very friendly and easy to talk to. I picked up many self-care tips from Rita and also from other women who attended the session."

—Pojanee D.

"I want you to also know that I have really felt a shift since the session in being willing to allow myself to do some of these things. I honestly think that having the validation from a group of women that self-care is not only okay but is crucial to my happiness and success in life. Validation is huge for me, having not gotten much of it throughout the majority of my life except for work I have done or 'accomplishments' I have had. I just had a funny thought...self-care is kind of like an extension of God's love for ourselves. It is that love that says you are worthy and deserving just because you are a living, breathing human being. I think that is another thing that has caused me to not do much in the way of self-care in the past. Because I am so hard on myself I never feel like I 'deserve' to do these things for myself. Hmmm...interesting to see the connections."

—Jennifer F.

"I like the one thing concept for self-care as it keeps it simple."

—Bernice Feaster,
Founder and Owner,
The Scholar Mom, LLC

"What Rita's self-care program has meant to me first and foremost is that it is ok to care about myself, to take the same care of myself as I do my family and pets and parents, and friends. To treat myself with the same care I would give to another. In my life I have spent so much time caring and scheduling the life of my family that I totally ignored myself.

"Rita's simple self-care impacted me the most when Rita spoke about caring for ourselves as essential in order to function fully. That it was ok and necessary to take care of our own needs. To listen to your emotional and physical needs before they start to crack and break. Rita gave me the green light to schedule time for myself. I especially love all the exercises I could do without having to grab a bag and go to a gym. I could be in a car line, at the grocery, cooking, etc. and there was an exercise Rita suggested that I could do. I also loved all the oils, and infusers. Rita has taught me that self-care doesn't have to be complicated or expensive. That I don't have to neglect my body and mind because a program is too complicated, pricey, demanding. Simple self-care tailored to my specific needs, challenges, life; and in this way I am able to stay committed to caring for myself because of the simplicity of Rita's program."

—Dina Feiden

"Dear Rita, The Light of Church Women's Conference was very meaningful to me and I want to thank you for participating as a speaker at that conference. Your words on 'Self-Care' *resonated to me and I decided that even if I couldn't run a marathon I could take one day at a time and do SOMETHING! My SOMETHING was to give up bacon! Bacon, for me is a huge comfort food* but I knew it was bad for me in so many ways. Whenever I have the urge to order a BLT or cook bacon on Sunday morning, I hear your voice very clearly reminding me that I just have to do SOMETHING. You helped me, and my blood pressure, more than you will ever know.

"Thanks so much Rita, and keep reminding folks that they can always do SOMETHING!"

—Jill Rajala

Simple Self-Care
Saved Me

Rita K. Garnto

Rita K. Garnto can be reached at rita@simpleselfcare.net or www.simpleselfcare.net

Published by Prominence Publishing www.prominencepublishing.com

Illustrations and Cover Graphics by Visual Caffeine.
www.visualcaffeine.com

ISBN: 978-1-988925-16-5

First Edition: January 2018

DEDICATION

To my loving and supportive husband. Thank you, Neal, for allowing me to fly, crash land, and keep on flying.

To my Dad for my adventurous soul.

To my Mom for my feisty spirit.

To my beautiful daughters for helping shape who I am today.

To Leann … you know, just 'cause.

TABLE OF CONTENTS

INTRODUCTION

Because of self-care, I can do what I do. Period. There is no other way to put it: Simple self-care has saved me in all aspects of life - mentally, emotionally, physically and spiritually. I am so excited to share with you what I have learned so far in this journey called "Life".

We all have our own journeys, and each is unique and special because it belongs to us. Just like no two people are alike, no two journeys are alike. I firmly believe because of this, we owe it to ourselves to claim our specialness, beauty, and uniqueness because it makes us who we are. Each and every one of us is a gift, but unfortunately, often times we don't see ourselves as a gift, rather, we see ourselves as *not good enough* and perhaps, as a disappointment and less than worthy.

I have so often struggled with low self-esteem and self-confidence issues through the years, especially as a teenager and then as a twenty-something, thirty-something, and even as a forty-something. As a result, I have devalued my own worth time and time again.

The amazing thing about life is that with each passing decade, I can see my self-value growing by leaps and bounds. The trick is to pay attention to life's lessons and keep learning from our failures. The only true failure is when you don't get back up after falling flat on your face. (Been there and done that over and over and over …)

Unfortunately, I know I am not alone in these struggles and that is part of the reason I am writing this book. Not only do I want to show you how easy is it to make your life more positive by changing just one thing, but I am hoping that through sharing my story and all its crazy challenges, you will see how important your story is. I want you to see what a beautiful gift you are.

It is time Ladies, to learn how to make your life better by simply putting yourself on the top of your to-do list. I will walk you through how to do this with simple self-care. I strongly suggest that you keep a journal, a notebook, or computer nearby to make notes of the things that resonate with you. Or, if you are like me, I highlight things in the book as I am reading it. This will be very helpful when you get to the part of the book where you start jotting down *your preferred* self-care on your way to discovering your one simple self-care key.

We are all born with our own set of circumstances - demographics, cultural, racial, sexual, financial - and what you decide to do with the circumstances of your journey is up to you. Do you become the victor or the victim? Do you use your journey to find your purpose to serve others or do you use it as a crutch and an excuse for not moving forward?

I have been alive now for just over half a century. (Boy, does that perspective make me sound old!) I have come to realize that no matter how you look at life, life can be hard and then, even harder at times. Life is full of challenges and full of brick walls to run into, go around, go under, or go over. Full of lessons and trials and tribulations. We can choose to grow or go stagnant.

Note: Pity parties are allowed for a little while, a couple of hours, half a day, or even a whole day, but then you have to get over it and figure out how to move on. Self-care can be such a great way to move forward after the pity party is over. I like to say … *time to put your big girl panties on and get over it.* More help, of course, with that later.

As I watch family members and family friends pass away, I am reminded of my own mortality and fragility. We truly only have one chance at this thing called "life" and what we do with our life is only a decision that each and every one of us can make. As I watch my two beautiful children grow up, I am reminded of this … that their lives are full of choices. I can arm them with lots of tools, information, love, and support, but I can *not* live their lives for them or make their choices for them, just like my Mom couldn't live my life for me. By picking up this book and starting to read it, you have already made a choice to take better care of yourself. Yay you!!

When it comes right down to it, you are the only one that will truly make the biggest difference in your life.

The media and our own culture often minimizes how important we all are and maximizes and fictionalizes "perfectionism". There is no such thing as the "perfect" body, "perfect" hair color, skin color, age, measurements - and the list goes on. We have been given what we have by our Creator and it is up to us to make the most of what we have, regardless of the shape of our hips or boobs, or how big or small our butts are. It's time to *own it* Ladies, and tell our inner bitches to take a hike! You deserve to be the best you can be.

There are times when I stumble and do not do the self-care things I should, and yes, I pay for those stumbles with extra aches and pains, unnecessary anxiety, increased emotional stress, and even increased irritability. To recover from this lack of self-care, I may need extra trips to my chiropractor and massage therapist, extra alone/me time, journaling, praying, or whatever will take me back to my good place. These blips of extra pain and physical, mental, spiritual, and emotional discomfort are reminders of how important it is that we take care of ourselves not only for our sake, but for the sakes of *all* those that rely on, love, and need us.

My two basic philosophies are: 1) keep it simple sweetie, and 2) do just one new thing, which I call *The Philosophy of One*. This book will explain the why's and the what's and the how's of these two simple concepts so that you will be able to take yourself from the bottom of your to-do list to the TOP with simple self-care effortlessly, and easily. That, my friend, is my promise to you!

Now, I know what you may be thinking, "How can something so simple actually work?" Well, stick with me because I am going to show you how. Unfortunately, our society has led us to believe in order to be successful, defined as losing weight, achieving your goals, feeling better, making lots of money or however you define it, we need to deprive ourselves and *fight* to attain our goal. We are led to believe that it must be hard and painful and miserable. NO! It doesn't. Self-care should provide you with joy, self-fulfillment, relaxation, relief and NOT deprivation, struggle, and denial. Self-care is about enjoying your life now and making it just a little easier to cope with what you are currently dealing with.

The book is set up in five sections. The first section is a basic introduction to self-care including the definitions of self-care and simple self-care and why I make a big distinction between the two. Section 2 gives you the down and dirty of why self-care is so very important to the quality of our health and lives. You will learn about the negative and serious effects stress can have on your health and well-being. You will also learn what is going on inside your body with each and every stress response and how this can impact your future health.

Section 3 is all about the process of finding *your* one simple self-care. I will walk you through the three steps to get you there. In section 4, we'll put all the pieces together while working through mental roadblocks you may run into. Section 5 gives you tools to help you to stay on track, and finally, section 6 sums it all up. A resource section is also included at the very end.

Ready. Set. Go.
Happy Self-Caring,

ACKNOWLEDGMENTS

My deepest gratitude to:

Cheale Villa for the kick in the hiney to get me started on the book and for bringing Sophie Self-Care to life as well as believing in me and all the support and love you have given me on this crazy journey of self-care. Thank you!

Halli Gomez for being my amazing mentor and editor with so much writing wisdom that made creating this book so much easier than it could have been. You are right … staring at the word counter doesn't make the number go up!

Melissa Baker, Jennifer E. Garnto, Ronnie Hamman, Ronnie Londner, Elaine Meertens-Cox, and Katja Wolf, my beta readers, for their time and very insightful comments and critiques. Thank you Ladies! Could not have done this without you.

To my family, friends, research subjects, Facebook friends, neighbors, and business associates that have shared their self-care journeys with me. Last, but in no way least, to Karen Preston, an extra hug, … "Who knew?!"

For we live by faith, not by sight.

~ 2 Corinthians 5:7

The Dragonfly

Often, I am asked, "Why the dragonfly?"

To make a long story, short … the dragonfly *found* me when I was just starting massage therapy school back in 2001. This simple dragonfly became my logo as a student massage therapist.

I later found out that dragonflies symbolize transformation and change (see quoted sources below), and are bringers of light. Wow! If that little dragonfly was not an accurate predictor of what was yet to come, I don't what could have been.

From that point in my life, my journey began to do a complete turnabout and it has led to wonderful, tragic, gut-wrenching, and inspiring monumental moments that have not only transformed, but completely changed my life.

As my life journey has evolved, so has my dragonfly companion. I love the little buddy that God has given me that serves as a reminder of the beautiful possibilities of life. Nothing is set in stone and through Faith, Love, and Perseverance, darkness in our lives can and will be overcome!

To summarize what dragonflies mean to me, they are a symbol of hope and light in a sometimes very dark world. By discovering and finding answers through self-awareness, self-love, and education, powerful change and positive transformation happens.

"The dragonfly symbolizes wisdom, change, transformation, light and adaptability in life. The dragonfly shows up in people's lives to remind them that they need to bring a lightness and a joy to their life."

-Reference.com

"The dragonfly, in almost every part of the world, symbolizes change and change in the perspective of self realization; and the kind of change that has its source in mental and emotional maturity and the understanding of the deeper **meaning** of life."

-Dragonfly-site.com

SECTION 1

INTRO TO SELF-CARE

A journey of a thousand miles begins with one single step.

~ Lao Tzu

Self-Care Defined

According to **dictionary.com**, self-care is a noun and it means *"care of the self without medical or other professional consultation."* To make this definition more useable, let's break it down into smaller "bits" and reword the definition to include the many aspects of *self* that we are made up of.

> *Self-care is any intentional action you take to care for your mental, emotional, physical, and spiritual health.*

Sounds easy enough, right?! But, in this day and age with instant access to all kinds of information at our fingertips, we can easily be inundated and overwhelmed. I know I am - frequently! Every day we receive insane amounts of new information via emails, tweets, texts, instagrams, research, and reports. What information is right for me? Which latest greatest product is best for me? How can I afford all this? What do I really need? Where the hell do I start? I'm drowning in information!! Ack!!

My hope with this book is to show you how to figure out *your* starting point. You will discover the *one* simple self-care that will help you embark on your self-care journey. For some reason, we women seem to think that we cannot just pick *one* thing, rather we need to take on two, three or five. The key word for this book is **one**. The goal is to simplify your search for the catalyst to begin your change and transformation.

The questions you will be able to answer by the end of the book are:

- Why should I do simple self-care?
- How do I figure out what is going to work for me?
- Where do I start?
- What do I start with?
- How do I stay on track?
- What tools will work for me?
- What are some common roadblocks I might run into?

Keep Life Simple

So, What the Heck is *Simple* Self-Care?

Life can be overwhelming. We have so much information thrown at us on a daily basis: emails, internet, TV programs, the latest and greatest news, discoveries, and fads. It just gets to be too much. I wanted to create a much more simplistic way to approach self-care. The answers to our questions do *not* need to be more complex in order to work. Rather, let's make life a little more e-a-s-y.

In this book, you will come to understand the difference between self-care and *simple* self-care. If you are looking for the latest and greatest workout or the latest news on how to lose weight with a new fad, this is not the book for you. I repeat, this is *not* the book for you.

This book is about finding the simple things that you can slide effortlessly into your day without the added stress and anxiety of trying to squeeze in *one more thing* into your already busy schedule.

The goal of this book is to start you on *your* path of transformation by finding the one simple self-care change you can make now without adding any stress or time commitments to your day. This one small change can and will act as a catalyst for the next change, and then the next change.

Please keep in mind that this is *not* an overnight process. You may not feel ready to make another simple self-care change for weeks or months and that is so OK! My own self-care and simple self-care routine has evolved over many years and continues to evolve as I get older and my body and my life changes.

It truly is a process. One of the women I interviewed during the writing of this book shared with me that her self-care transformation started with focusing on only one change the first year. Then she made another change in the second year of her journey, and then a third change in her third year. Now she is in an amazing new place in her life. Not only has she lost over 160 pounds in those three years and is walking two to three miles daily, but her self-confidence, well-being, and zest for life have all grown immensely. Whenever I see her walking, she has a big smile on her face and she glows! The biggest takeaways for me from her story are (a) her process started with one change, (b) she has been consistent and patient, and (c) it takes time. It is a process, indeed.

Whether you make one change today and then feel ready for the next change next week or next month or next year, it does not matter. This is about consistency, patience, and faith. This is very much about *you* and what works for *you*. I cannot stress this enough … this is all about you, my friend! I know, I know, you don't get to hear that very often so it is about time that someone makes it about you.

Back to our definition of self-care: **any intentional action you take to care for your mental, emotional, physical, and spiritual health.** By using this definition, you could probably write down 10, 20, or maybe 30 different self-care things that you could do. Most of them would most likely take a time commitment on your part you may not be ready to invest in. Maybe you just do not have any more time to devote to anything else right now. If you are feeling a time crunch, this book is definitely for you!

Please do not misinterpret what I am saying. Self-care is important and very crucial to our well-being. The problem I am addressing is when life gets so busy and you have to choose between getting all your things done and doing your self-care. Inevitably, your self-care will be the first thing to fall off your to-do list. This book offers you *more* choices that will take virtually no extra time so you can put yourself on the top of your to-do list and still take care of the things you need to take care of.

The word *simple* refers to something being easy to understand, not complex nor complicated. By putting the two definitions together, simple self-care becomes *an intentional self-care action that is easy, not rocket-science nor complex, and will effortlessly slide into your day.*

By taking into account your busy life, the simple self-care piece should *flow* into your busy schedule as opposed to being *squeezed* in somewhere. My simple self-care concept is based on the ability to slide your self-care into various moments of your day without any great effort. The more effort, willpower, and fight it takes to do your self-care, the greater the energy waste, both physically and mentally, and greater the increase in stress and anxiety levels.

Let me give you an example. In the past, I have really enjoyed going to the gym to workout. I'm a gym-rat from the 80's and have always found it a great way to stay in shape and keep my anxiety and stress levels down. And yet these days, I often struggle with making the time to go regularly to the gym. Yes, working out at the gym can be great self-care and yes, it is important to my well-being; however, if I can't find the energy or time to go, what is the point of trying to force myself to go or feel guilty if I don't go? That just seems counterproductive. So, with the simple self-care approach I decide to walk my dogs in my neighborhood and do planks, stretches, and crunches at home. It's quicker, easier, and less effort and for now, fits into my life better than the gym. The biggest piece is that I am keeping my stress level down by listening to my body and being more *user-friendly* to me!

An important tidbit of information which you may not realize is when you allow your stress level to increase, regardless of whether it's from mental, physical, or emotional factors, your body enters the *fight or flight* mode. This mode triggers a lot of changes inside our bodies and over time, can often lead to some serious health issues. More on all that stress stuff a little later.

Even if your stress level didn't increase and your body does not experience the stress response, think of all the energy you have just wasted thinking about doing self-care that does not (a) resonate with you and (b) doesn't fit into your life right now. On top of all that, you have wasted energy on feeling guilty and then wasted even more energy on beating yourself up about it! Sound familiar?

Whew!! I'm making myself tired just thinking about all that energy waste! Wouldn't it make sense and be more logical to use all that energy on something more fun and productive?!

Before I give you an example of simple self-care, let me introduce you to Sophie Self-Care. Sophie is a working woman. She's busy and exhausted. She's every woman. But, she's learned a big lesson this year: she can't pour from an empty cup. Something we all often realize too late. So, she's filling up with simple self-care tactics and wants to be an inspiration for you to do the same. Change one thing and change your entire life. Think of Sophie as your guide to help you learn more about simple self-care and how easy it is to incorporate it into your daily life!

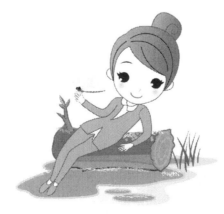

Throughout the book, she will be demonstrating the different simple self-care choices. If you are still not sure what I mean by *simple* self-care, here is an example:

Give Yourself a Hug: *Before getting out of bed in the morning, slowly bring your knees towards your chest, hold, and take a few slow, deep breaths. This movement gently stretches your mid and lower back muscles along with your glutes. In essence, this "wakes up" your lower back before getting out of bed, thereby helping reduce the muscle strain on your lower back.*

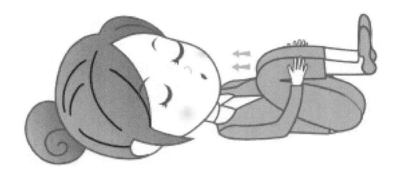

Now let me be perfectly honest and upfront with you … doing this gentle stretch every morning and maybe at bedtime is not a guarantee that you'll never have any back pain. However, it is a piece of simple self-care that is not rocket science, not complicated, is easy, and can effortlessly slide into your day. And yes, it will help reduce back discomfort and pain. By doing this simple stretch, you have taken yourself from the bottom of your to-do list to the top! YAY you! That, my dear, is what simple self-care is all about!

This is just one example of many that I will be presenting to you in a later chapter called *All Kinds of Simple Self-Care.* It continues to amaze me time and time again how just *one* simple variation to your routine can be the beginning of amazing transformation and positive change.

But what changes are <u>you</u> going to make?

My Story

Without simple self-care, I would not be doing what I do today. I know in my heart that both self-care and simple self-care have truly saved my life. So, what was the turning point in my life that the need for *simplifying* my self-care started to become glaringly obvious? Have you ever run into, figuratively speaking, of course, a brick wall? Have you ever reached a point where the thought of moving forward was too much effort and you just felt lost or maybe felt like the walls were collapsing in on you?

I have.

To help you get a better understanding of why I do what I do, here is part of my story. This story contains all the aspects of the self-care definition. I have struggled at times both mentally and emotionally with anxiety and depression. Physically, I continue to face many challenges from, not only a strong family history of osteoarthritis, but also from my own diagnoses of osteoarthritis in my knees, back, and neck. And finally, learning to rely on Faith and trusting in God has helped me grow in leaps and bounds spiritually by giving me the strength to continue to move forward in my journey in a positive frame of mind.

This part of my story deals with my struggles with infertility including four miscarriages, and a three-year adoption roller coaster ride ending in the adoption of our two beautiful daughters.

Brick Wall #1

It was a beautiful July morning with not a cloud in the sky. I clearly remember the beautiful sunshine and warmth from the sun that streamed into our kitchen. It was not too humid yet and for that, I was thankful. My girls, two and four at the time, and I were in the kitchen finishing up breakfast. We had just become a new family 6 months earlier and wow, was it a tough transition. Motherhood and parenting was a lot harder than I ever thought it would be. Looking back, good thing we didn't know how tough our parenthood journey was going to be!

One of the girls said or did something and I became frustrated. Realizing that I was almost at my breaking point, I headed out the back door to the deck telling the girls, "I need a Mommy moment".

I sat down on a deck chair and started to cry. As all kinds of thoughts swirled in my head, I began crying harder. Who was I as a Mom? Where has my old life gone? Wasn't it so much easier when it was just Neal and I alone? My massage business! What is going to happen to my massage business and my clients now that I can't fully engage and see all the clients I want. Oh my God, I am so, so tired. I'm such a crappy Mom. I yell too much. I'm not sure that I even like these little girls right now. Will I ever love them? Will they ever love me? Why don't they listen to me? What if they don't love me back?

The thoughts in my head don't stop moving.

And Neal. Who is he as a Dad? I'm seeing all sorts of sides of him and of me that I didn't know existed. It is frightening. I'm not sure I even like some of those sides. I can't take this. The stress. The emotions. The screaming. The tantrums. What have we done? Where do we go from here? Stop your screaming! Stop arguing with me! Stop saying your birth mom was better than me because her knees didn't hurt her. Stop telling me you hate this family. Stop pushing me away and then clinging to me. Love me. Hug me. Be my daughters. Stop the conflict. Where did the peace go in our house? The routine? The calmness? The tranquility?

Even our dogs notice the huge changes in our house. Our one dog that never wanted to be outside, begs to go out all the time now when the screaming starts. I don't know how to fix this. Dear Lord, please help us. I need strength. I can't take it anymore. I want to run away. My friends don't understand. "You wanted this," is what I hear from some of them. What have we done? Who have I become? I don't like who I am right now. How can I like anyone else? Oh my God, what is happening to us? To me? I need help! I can't do this anymore!!

As I sat sobbing on the deck with all these thoughts swirling in my head, I suddenly look up and see my youngest daughter staring at me.. She turned without a word, walked inside, and then reappeared with her sister. Now they were both standing looking at me, unsure of what to do, as the tears continued to roll down my face. My youngest pointed at me and said, "Mommy sad! Mommy sad!" Maybe on some level, it was meant to reassure me that they were aware I was crying but I just started to cry harder. I. Could. Not. Stop. Crying. Someone. Help me. Please!

A short while later, I called my husband sobbing and he rushed home. His presence brought me some degree of comfort and support and the tears stopped … for now. Later, on the phone with my doctor's office as I was making an appointment with the receptionist, the tears erupted and started flowing … again. How embarrassing, I thought. Thank goodness the receptionist was very understanding and comforting and this was probably not the first time she had a crying woman on the other end of the phone.

A little while later sitting in the doctor's office, I was seemingly composed until my doctor walked in. Here we go again … more tears and sobbing. I felt so horrible as my life was surely spinning out of control, or so I thought.

After a long, supportive, and comforting conversation, Dr. G. Weidner handed me a prescription. His words to me were, "This prescription is going to help, BUT what changes are you going to make?"

My thoughts raced. I thought, Pardon? What do you mean what am *I going to* change about my situation? Isn't this the solution right here on this piece of paper - the magic pill that makes it all go away? What? You want me to be accountable. Hmmm, never thought of that. You mean I actually have some control over my life? You mean that I can actually control some of this shit that is going on? You mean I can make choices that can positively effect my life even with all this stress and turmoil? Wow! Who knew?!

Little did he realize his question would cause me to actively seek solutions through self-care and then later, simple self-care, to help me deal with the stress of my life. Little did he realize his question that day would trigger the slow evolution of the concepts of *simple self-care* and the *philosophy of one*.

Little did he realize that he had empowered me with those simple words. From that point, my self-care journey took a sharp turn and I started being more aware of my limitations which included my time constraints, my responsibilities, and my financial situation. I then started looking at the self-care choices that would fit into my life and ones that I was physically able to do. I started asking myself what kind of self-care is important to me, what would feed my spirit, and what would help me control my stress. The simple self-care concept slowly emerged. However, it would take me several years to fully embrace the *power of simple* along with the idea of making just one change at a time.

That morning when I had unraveled before my daughters was me finally running into brick wall #1. This was the moment I realized that I was the only one that could take control and do something about the stress in my life. This was the time for increased self-awareness and self-care. Not only did my quality of life, health, and sanity depend on it, but also my husband, daughters, parents, friends, and clients.

Even with this great epiphany, little did I know that within the next two and half years, I would have to deal with two more catastrophic life-changing events. You know, it really is good we don't know what lies ahead of us in our journeys.

Brick Wall #2

A year and a half later in August 2010, my Mom died very unexpectedly and suddenly. I had just spoken to her three times on the phone the day before. I thank the Lord that they were all good conversations and that I told her I loved her.

She was only 75 years old and she passed away from a massive heart attack, leaving my 81 year old Dad alone … 3000 miles away and not in great health. I now assumed the role of caretaker of an aging parent.

The next year involved five trips to my hometown, Kamloops, British Columbia, helping my Dad adjust to losing his wife of 52 years. The first trip was when my Mom had passed in August for her funeral. The second trip was shortly thereafter for a pre-planned and already paid trip for my Dad's birthday in September. As a matter of fact, those last conversations with my Mom were about that surprise birthday trip. Trip number three came a few months later at Christmastime. Neal, the girls, and I joined my brother and his family at my Dad's for the first Christmas without Mom. The next two trips were in June and September of 2011. On that last trip, as my youngest daughter and I were getting our luggage, I developed a pain in my left upper back. Not thinking much of it and thinking it was probably a strained muscle, I continued to do my self-care and take Advil to try to numb the pain.

Eight weeks later and fully immersed back into my life, I was still living in excruciating pain and had resorted to eating ibuprofen like candy for pain management. (Note: This is NOT a good idea nor was this one of my better decisions as taking large doses of ibuprofen can lead to liver and kidney failure. Rest assured, I received a well-deserved and extensive lecture from my surgeon regarding this unsafe practice.) When I finally received the MRI results, after having to convince the nurse practitioner that I really needed one, the verdict was in. The disc between vertebrae C6 and C7 in my neck had ruptured and was compressing the nerves in the left side of my neck. This was not good! Not until I met with the surgeon later that week did I discover that my left arm was also noticeably weaker than my right arm. Double not-good!! Surgery was scheduled for three weeks later.

The surgery went well and my recovery went smoothly. My cervical spine now has three fused vertebrae (C5, 6, & 7) to prevent further degeneration and to provide support for this part of my spine. I am also sporting a titanium plate, 3 screws, and a couple of cadaver bones. Oh, and a very pretty, hardly noticeable scar. Thank you Dr. T!

My disc rupture was brick wall # 2 and I knew that I needed to make even more changes in my life. I was literally killing myself and my body was screaming at me. I took eight weeks off from my massage practice and when I did go back it was to a new part-time schedule so I could take better care of myself and my family.

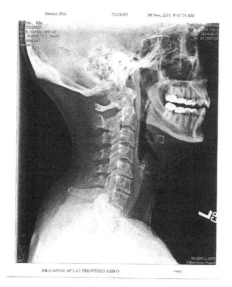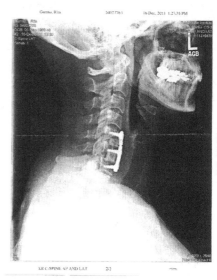

These are xrays of my neck before (left) and after (right) the surgery. Notice the lovely hardware I am now sporting.

Remember that any of the self-care or simple self-care choices you make are for you and you alone. If it can't fit into your life right now or you don't have the money, time, or desire, then it is *not* the right choice. Much more on that later.

In case you are wondering what self-care changes I have made after my first brick wall encounter, here are some of them. My first change was going back to the gym to workout once a week by getting up at 5 AM and being home by 7 AM so Neal could go to work. Yes, I got up that early *but* it was only one day a week so I was able to convince myself to get up. Honestly, it was not easy most days.

We continued with *quiet time* in the afternoons so I could read and chill out – it really was more for me than the kids. The girls continued with part-time childcare during the times I worked so there was no real extra downtime for me without the girls. I journaled, did acupuncture regularly, got massages regularly, continued with chiropractic care, and tried to focus on eating "cleaner" with more fruits and vegetables. I continued with counseling, my prescribed medication, and worked with a psychiatrist for a while.

Now, the self-care and simple self-care that I continue to do on a regular basis includes: journaling, reading, walks with my dogs, quiet time, Mommy time, ice wraps for aching joints, supplements, stretching, taekwando, working out at the gym, using a flaxseed neck wrap for tight neck, shoulder, and upper back muscles, aromatherapy, Epsom salt baths, favorite music playlists, socializing, talking, and sharing with friends, deep breathing, and practicing self-awareness, self- acceptance, gratitude, and self-love. Please do not let my list overwhelm or intimidate you ... I have been at this for a very long time. My self-care journey started in my teens with journaling and exercise as a way to cope with my anxiety and tumultuous emotions. At the time, I did not realize I was doing self- care as I was just trying to cope with being a teenager. Reality check: I have been at this self-care thing for over 40 years! Yes, it is a process and you have to start somewhere and it is never too late!

Just a quick comment about medication. I strongly believe there is a place in our lives that medication is warranted and effective (especially in cases of chemical imbalances and diagnosed mental health issues). I do not believe, however, that they are the *only* solution, ever. Medication can act as a bridge during the stressful times when we need extra biochemical support, and self-care is a must to go along with that. Good mental and emotional health requires a multi-prong approach. Yes, perhaps, too many people are on medications or maybe they are too easily prescribed because, I think, as a society we look for the easy way out. We want instant gratification without much work or effort . This attitude, my friend, will not help you evolve and become the best woman you are meant to be.

I cannot thank Dr. G. Weidner enough for not only prescribing the medication I needed at the time, but also challenging me to look at other options for taking care of myself. Is it easy? Hell no, but these challenges and choices and changes we make transform us into wiser, more beautiful, and healthier women that can serve our purpose while taking care not only of ourselves, but also those that depend on us.

> *Self-care is not about self-indulgence.*
> *It is about self-preservation.*
> ~ *Audrey Lorde*

My Passion and Mission

My passion is to make a difference in other women's lives. I hope to inspire by sharing the reality, the good, the bad, and the ugly of my life. Yes, it may sound like a cliché to you, however, I feel this purpose, this passion, is pushing me to write this book and reach out to women everywhere.

My mission is to show women how to put themselves on the top of their to-do lists with simple self-care. It's that basic, well, simple. My hopes are to create support systems and communities where women can feel safe, nurtured, and understood. Yes, all our stories are different, but our feelings and emotions are all very similar.

The belief that *"everything happens for a reason – there is no coincidence"* shapes my reality. I did not go through all this crap just for my own personal growth or just to improve my life. My message of survival, having faith, and the ability to turn your life around with *one* simple self-care change needs to be heard!

There are women and men everywhere that think they are alone as they deal with their struggles. Your life story may be worded slightly different, but *you* are not alone! Others, including me, have gone through and dealt with similar, if not the same things, you are dealing with. I am here to tell you that you are not alone!

Feeling a part of a community that is loving and supportive can make all the difference in your life. It has shaped my life the last few years and I can just not stress the importance enough. I can confidently say that *I have a tribe!* I am so very grateful and blessed to have these many strong women and men in my life. Thank you!

Too Much Information

The way I see it is that I have been blessed with the personality trait of not being afraid to stand up in a room full of people and share. I am not afraid to let others see inside of me and see my vulnerability. This was not always case, though. Until recently, I used to consider this sharing as a faulty personality trait and would often hear, "TMI*, Rita! TMI*!", and be accused of sharing too much personal information. And then, I would often feel remorse and guilt after I had shared a story or personal information, but could never seem to stop sharing the next time round.

(*too much information)

Then I discovered **Brené Brown**, the Vulnerability Researcher. Love her message! After watching her 2010 TED talk, *The Power of Vulnerability*, I was able to begin to make sense of what I had been thinking was this bad personality trait. Brené, as a researcher, studied how people make relationships and one of her conclusions was that *"being vulnerable allows us to connect and create relationships"*. After listening to her TED talk, I began to understand that by making myself vulnerable with my information sharing was how I was connecting and creating bonds with others. The ones that criticized me were just not ready to connect.

Thank you Brené!!! (I hope to meet you someday!) For more information about her books, please see the resource section at the end of this book.

Choices ... We All Have Them

The importance of choices. How important are the choices we make? Do we ever stop and think about all the choices we have in front of us and the multitude of choices we make every day? It has become painfully obvious, especially now that I am a parent, that all choices lead to consequences. These consequences can be good, bad, or just downright ugly. I preach to my children constantly about the choices they have available to them and the consequences attached. I want my children growing up thinking and being aware of their actions, and being responsible and accountable to themselves and others.

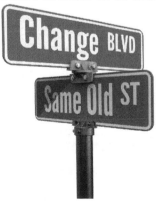

Now, I didn't grow up with this way of parenting. As I was growing up, it was never pointed out to me that my choices had consequences and in fact, a lot of my choices were made *for* me by someone else. I learned to not really have an opinion or really understand that I had the right to make my own choices and not be swayed by others. Believe it or not, even in my 30's, I still had problems with making some of my own choices without asking someone else's opinion. Another life lesson I had to learn.

Think about how many hundreds, or thousands of choices we make every day. Do you ever stop to think how about each little choice impacts our lives? I sure don't. Just by deciding to take one road route home over another can save you from accident or put you in harm's way.

OK. This way of thinking is not meant to increase your anxiety level because after re-reading those lines, my anxiety level surged just a little. My point is that this way of thinking is really about the *awareness* of the choices we have available to us. Repeat after me: I always have a choice.

The choice I want to talk specifically about now is the choice to start *making yourself a priority with daily simple self-care*. Once we have decided to do something by making a choice to do it, it is not always easy to stick with that choice. We falter, we forget, we get complacent, or we just simply choose not to continue because of some excuse, fear, or ugly gremlin rearing its nasty little head.

This is life. Life is dynamic and has ups and downs and all-arounds. Life is good, bad, and sometimes just OK. Life flows and it is a process. There is no specific end-point or goal to be reached. It's a journey that we are on and this journey can and will take us to all kinds of places where we never dreamed of going and in some cases, never, ever wanted to go.

The simple fact that you are reading this book, tells me that you have already made the choice to take better care of yourself with simple self-care and that you are ready to make some new choices and are open to new ways of looking at things in your life. This, my friend, is what I call a "YAY ME!" moment. Embrace it and pat yourself on the back! And, thank you! Writing this book is part of my purpose to serve and I am so grateful and blessed to have you as one of my readers.

THE DOWN AND DIRTY OF STRESS

With awareness comes motivation and positive change.

Your Health History Matters

Simple self-care is a powerful neutralizer of the negative effects of stress. Before, I think, you can truly understand why that is, you need to know what is happening in your body during a stress response and how that will impact your future health and well-being. I am hoping that by providing this information in the next part of this book in an easy and understandable format, you may find nuggets of information that will Strengthen your *a-ha moment* and motivation.

When it comes right down to it, if the stress response continues to occur over, over, over, and over again without sufficient relief your body, mind, and spirit can and will unequivocally suffer. I believe that accumulative negative stress without sufficient simple self-care can be deadly.

As I mentioned earlier, my Mom passed away in 2010 at the age of 75 from a massive heart attack. I attribute her premature passing to the amount of negative stress she had been under for a long period of time coupled with her lack of sufficient self-care and a strong history of heart disease. She often put the care of others before the care of herself and I got the sense that she felt like she didn't deserve to take more time for herself which was so very unfortunate. Maybe that was a generational frame of mind or something she carried over from her childhood and upbringing.

For me, the stark reality of her passing is not only that I lost my Mom too soon, but that I have a strong family history of heart disease. To view this in a more positive light, I can use this piece of information as one of my *a-ha moments* to fuel my motivation to keep my blood pressure in a normal range, keep my weight down, and be aware of good, healthy eating habits along with maintaining my simple self-care practice.

You cannot change your family health history, but knowledge is power and you can use that information to help fuel your resolve to take action and work towards a healthier you.

Take a brief moment to make note of any major health issues that run in your family.

_____

_____

_____

_____

_____

_____

Now, use this information as a way to create an *a-ha Moment* for you.

Because my family health history includes _____

_____

_____,

I **want** *and* **need** *to take better care of myself.*

God may forgive your sins, but your nervous system won't.

~ Alfred Korzybski

Your Nervous System

Before we delve into what *the Down and Dirty of Stress* is all about, let's take a moment to talk about your body, specifically, your nervous system.

The definition of the nervous system according to **http://kidshealth. org/en/kids/word-nervous-system.html** states:

The nervous system controls everything you do, including breathing, walking, thinking, and feeling. This system is made up of your <u>brain</u>, spinal cord, and all the nerves of your body.

It's Not Just a Brain

The brain is the center of all your thoughts, the origin of control of all body movement, and the interpreter of all the information that is gathered and transmitted by the peripheral nerves. As complex and sophisticated as your brain is, it still needs this link to the outside world, via the peripheral nerves, or it would be utterly useless. All the information your peripheral nerves gather and send back to your brain allows your brain to know what is going on in your surroundings and environment to keep us safe, functioning, and alive.

Basically, your nervous system consists of two major parts: (1) the central nervous system, CNS, and (2) the peripheral nervous system, PNS. The CNS consists of the brain and the spinal cord while the PNS consists of all the nerves *outside* of the brain and spinal cord. The peripheral nerves travel to the rest of your body including your extremities, internal organs, skin, and so on to provide the brain with lots of information about what is happening in all these areas.

Another way to look at this division between the central and peripheral nervous systems is to imagine your brain and spinal cord as the *main train station* where all the trains, the peripheral nerves, either start or end their journeys.

The peripheral nerves that make up the peripheral nervous system also consist of two different types. The first type are called the *sensory* nerves. These nerves detect sensations such as changes in temperature (skin), light (retina of the eye), mechanical forces (touch, pressure, vibration, stretch, itch), the presence of chemicals (molecules tasted or smelled), and pain (caused by potentially damaging stimuli). Another way to think of them is to call them the *feeling* nerves. They provide the brain information regarding our surroundings and environment.

The second type of nerves are called the *motor* nerves. These control, you guessed it, movement. The brain sends signals along these nerves when we want or need to have some type of movement or motion. Without these nerves, we would literally be paralyzed and be at the mercy of the world.

Here's an example of how these two types of nerve networks function together. Let's say you touch a hot stove. The immediate response is a signal traveling from your hand to your brain saying, "Oh! Really HOT!" These are the sensory nerves at work. When this message reaches the brain, it sends a message back to the hand via the motor nerves saying, "Move your hand NOW!" You move your hand and hopefully do not sustain any major burns. As you well know and I am sure, have experienced, this process happens in mere nanoseconds, thank God! We need both these type nerves to function safely in our lives.

Motor Nerves

Now, let's talk more about the motor nerves. The motor nerves are also divided into two groups. These groups are called voluntary and involuntary motor nerves. Voluntary, as in, I want to pick up that glass of water, and involuntary, as in, my pancreas just released some insulin without me thinking about it because of the chocolate I just ate.

Let's just take a brief moment and think about ALL the involuntary functions our bodies perform without us even realizing it: breathing, heart beating, hormone secreting, digesting, and the list goes on. Our bodies really are amazing creations and often, we forget how truly blessed we are. How often do you thank your body for all the wonderful things it does without you asking it? How about some self-love for a moment? Big hug!

Next, let's talk about the involuntary nervous system. You guessed it! It is also divided into two groups. Bear with me … almost done! This is where we get into the nitty gritty of the stress response.

This involuntary nervous system is the part of the nervous system that has to do with stress and relaxation and is called the autonomic nervous system, or ANS. Autonomic as in automatic. Again, no thought about triggering a response because it just happens.

Autonomic Nervous System

Some background info about the ANS. This part of the nervous system controls and regulates the functions of your internal organs including your heart, intestines, stomach, liver, and pancreas. Since the ANS is part of the peripheral nervous system motor nerves, it also controls some of the muscles within the body. You may not have realized that these places on your body even had muscles. Ever wonder how goosebumps were created? When the muscles around the hair follicles contract, ta-da … goosebumps. Your blood pressure is controlled by the muscles in the walls of your blood vessels and the amount of light allowed to enter your eye is controlled by the muscles of your eye. Again, these are all controlled by the ANS and happen automatically … no conscious thought required.

The ANS also regulates the glandular systems in your body including the power houses: the adrenals which produce adrenalin and cortisol, the thyroid which plays a major role in the metabolism, growth and maturation of the human body, and the pituitary gland which is often considered the *master* gland.

As mentioned above, because the ANS functions involuntarily and reflexively, we are often unaware of the ANS doing its thing. For example, when you step outside into the sunlight, you are not aware of your pupils getting smaller because of the extreme brightness or you are not consciously aware of your heart rate increasing and muscles tensing when you see a car veer into your lane. This is the ANS working its magic!

Thank you for staying with me! All this information brings us closer to the down and dirty details of stress.

The ANS is extremely important in two situations: (1) emergency situations when you are in danger and need to fight or run away to save your life, and (2) nonemergency situations so you can rest, digest, recover, and recharge. Because the body's response to these different situations is vital to our survival, we have a specific part of the nervous system controlling what happens in each of these situations.

In emergency life and death situations, as well as when we are stressed or startled, the **sympathetic** nervous system is activated. A much more common name for this part of the nervous system, which you are probably very familiar with, is the *fight or flight* response.

For our bodies to maintain a healthy balance, there must exist a second part to the ANS that will help us rest, digest, recover, and recharge from real or perceived emergency situations. This part of the nervous system's function is essentially opposite to that of *fight or flight*. This other part of the nervous system is activated when we are calm and relaxed and is controlled by the **parasympathetic** nervous system. From now on, this will be known as the *resting and digesting* response.

On the next page is a flow chart that I have created to help you understand the progression of the divisions of our nervous system. The area I will be focusing on for the rest of the chapter is the last section entitled *Involuntary ANS*.

I hope it helps to give you a visual and ultimately, better understanding. No worries, no quiz at the end of this chapter!

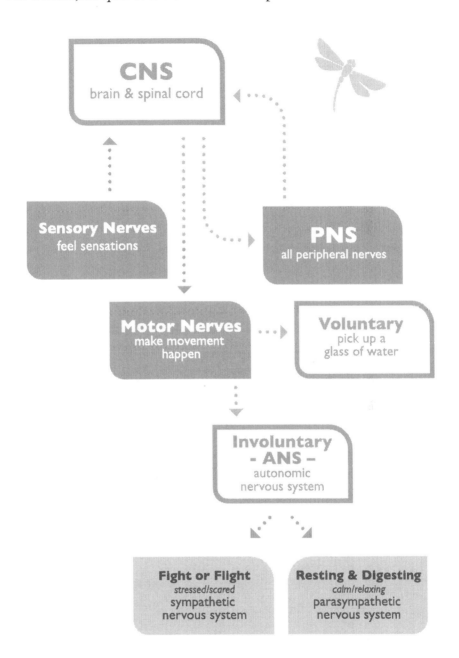

Dear Stress, Let's break up.

Defining Stress

STRESS can be defined as a biological (body) and psychological (mind) response that we experience when we encounter a threat and we feel we do not have enough resources to handle it. In other words, we enter a state of mental, physical, and emotional tension resulting from a threat, adverse, or demanding circumstance, real or perceived..

The STRESSOR, the *thing* causing the stress, is commonly called the trigger because it activates or triggers the stress response. We perceive this trigger as a threat and it creates the mental, physical, and emotional tension we feel within our bodies. The stressor can literally be any event, set of conditions, environment, or situation and doesn't matter if it is real or imagined. Examples of stressors include anything from a car driving towards you in your lane to facing a work deadline to your child having a tantrum in the middle of the grocery store aisle to spilling your coffee all over the kitchen floor. Some of these examples are not life and death, but your brain and body do not know the difference and will respond in a similar manner to each stressful situation.

Whatever your body perceives as a threat will trigger what is called the STRESS RESPONSE. Because your brain thinks you may not have enough resources to deal with a particular situation, additional resources are provided. These resources come in the form of extra energy, strength, and stamina and are created by the activation of the *fight or flight* response. Keep in mind this part of our nervous system works automatically and involuntarily, responding to your stress levels. Even without a conscious thought or action, we will experience the stress response.

Pause for a moment and consider that last sentence. We do not have to have a conscious thought or make a conscious effort for our bodies to react like we are facing a life and death situation. Hmmmm … so every time I experience road rage, my body is reacting like my life is in danger. Same response when I am running late for work or yelling at the kids. That doesn't sound very healthy. It's not ... stay tuned.

STRESS OVERLOAD happens when daily stressors become overwhelming and you, or even others, start to notice physical, emotional, and/or behavioral changes in you. This can happen if the stress you experience is caused by a very intense stressor such death of a loved one, divorce, or loss of a job, or if the stressors continue over a long period of time. This can include dealing with chronic health issues or long-term care of a sick or elderly family member. Stress overload can also manifest as a feeling of being very overwhelmed or feeling like your life is spinning out of control.

We all have a very *personalized* stress response to our stressors. This personalized response is dependent on the following four factors: (1) your previous exposure to the stressor, (2) your perception of the stressor, (3) your experience with the stressor, and (4) the healthy coping skills you have in place.

I find the personalized stress response so fascinating because the same stressor can create varying levels of stress in different people based on your past exposure, perception, experience, and coping skills.

A great example: you lose your job. Person A has experienced job loss before and has learned to be prepared by creating an emergency fund savings account. So, Person A has been saving money, planning for this job loss, and is honestly ready for a job change. Their stress reaction would be *very* different from Person B who was not expecting to get laid off and this job was the only source of income for the Person B's family. Same stressor, but different perceptions and experiences will create a much different stress response.

Another good example would be public speaking. I have no problem getting up in front of people to speak and have done it many times, but my husband not so much. Therefore, his stress reaction is much greater than mine when asked to speak in front of a group.

I stress about stress before there's even stress to stress about. Then I stress about stressing over stress that doesn't need to be stressed about. It's stressful.

What's Really Going On

Remember earlier, we talked about our autonomic nervous system and how it controls our glandular systems in our bodies. When we experience the stress response, the *fight or flight* part of our autonomic nervous system kicks in and releases the stress hormones adrenalin and cortisol. The release of these hormones causes the following to occur in your body systems: your heart rate increases, blood pressure increases, breathing rate increases, blood sugar levels increase, blood flow to your digestive tract decreases, and your immune response decreases. Here is a chart summarizing the changes that occur during the stress response.

SUMMARY of the STRESS RESPONSE:

__↑__ **Heart Rate**   __↑__ **Blood Pressure**

__↑__ **Breathing Rate**   __↑__ **Blood Sugar**

__↓__ **Blood Flow to Digestive Tract**

__↓__ **Immunity**

Why Stress Happens

Through much of human history, our ancestors have had to deal with extreme life and death situations. These dangers included wild animals, invading tribes, environmental extremes, and food scarcity. The stress response gave our ancestors' bodies the extra resources to deal with these dangers by providing the extra energy, strength, and stamina to either literally defend oneself (fight) or flee (flight).

When the stress reaction occurs, the increase in heart rate, blood pressure, and breathing rate create an increased amount of oxygen in the blood stream being delivered faster throughout the body. This, along with the increased amounts of sugar in the blood, provide the extra fuel needed by the body during the stress response. The blood flow to the digestive tract is decreased because the immediate digestion of the food within the digestive tract is not crucial to your immediate survival. In other words, having your body continue to digest that grilled chicken salad you had for lunch is not going to help you get out of a burning car. This diverted blood flow is better utilized by muscles to help you get out of the burning car. The immune system is also **not** a priority during this stressful time. Let's face it, if we don't survive this life and death situation, we won't need an immune system in the future. So again, energy is taken away from our immune system and our immune response decreases.

Another interesting fact is your higher level of thinking – the critical decision making – is also *shut off* during stressful times. Blood flow to the brain is diverted to areas that are most crucial for your survival. When you are in the heat of your crisis situation, you are functioning on adrenalin to survive. In this state, you can run faster, move quicker, be stronger, have longer stamina and frankly, don't need to logically think. We have all heard, I'm sure, about the Mom who lifts a car off of her trapped toddler. This stress reaction is the reason why she was able to do that.

The Good News

The *good* news about the stress reaction is that it forces us to adapt and overcome adversity. This stress response keeps us alive and coping. We need stress for personal development and growth. Not all stress is bad. There is also *good* stress such as getting engaged or finding out you are pregnant or getting a promotion.

As stated in the article, *What is Stress?*, *https://www.stress.org/what-is-stress*, "… stress can be helpful and good when it motivates people to accomplish more. … increased stress results in increased productivity – up to a point, …"

The Bad News

OK, now the bad news about the stress reaction. It has not changed as the human race and our lifestyles have evolved. What this means is that even though we don't necessarily need this extreme stress response to deal with our daily stressors, our bodies often interpret the stress we feel as a life and death situation. In other words, whenever we face a work deadline, child's tantrum, spilling our coffee, financial issues, or whatever situation we may perceive as stressful, even though it is *not* a life and death situation, our bodies react like it is.

To compound the problem further, we no longer have the same coping mechanisms in place in our everyday lives that our ancestors did. For the most part, our ancestors led a very physical life with *forced periods* of relaxation. Forced periods of relaxation happened when the sun set. No electricity meant no sources of light other than fire. When the sun went down, the day was done. We gathered in our caves, log cabins, or tents with our tribe and families, cooked and ate our meals, and allowed our bodies to wind down in preparation for sleep.

In addition to the daily periods of forced relaxation, consistent physical labor – plowing the fields, gathering food, hunting - would allow the working muscles to consume the excess amount blood sugar, an effect of the stress reaction, for fuel on a consistent basis. Physical activity helps blood sugar levels return back to normal after a stressful encounter. Also, after physical exertion, blood pressure, heart rate, and breathing rate typically return to normal levels as well. All these activities helped counteract the effects of the stress reactions.

Look at us today. Plugged in 24/7 … day and night. Because of technology, we are no longer *forced* to put our work away, but rather can work on and on and on. Now, it becomes a much bigger self-regulated lifestyle, that we need, with effective boundaries. Awareness of what our minds, bodies, and spirits need, I think, has become more important than ever.

The truth of the matter is … if we do not have effective self-care and coping skills in place, the repetitive stress response is going to impede our quality of health and eventually, kill us!

It's not the load that breaks you down, it's the way you carry it.
~ Lou Holtz

How Stressed Are You?

The peak of stress overload (aka running into *your* brick wall) differs for each of us. Being sensitive to the early warning signs and symptoms that may suggest an impeding stress overload, is super important. The signs and symptoms differ for each of us and can be so subtle that they are often ignored until it is too late. Not infrequently, others are more aware you may be headed for trouble before you are. Check in with a close friend to see if she has noticed any changes related to stress in your behavior. See the following list for signs and symptoms of stress overload. Make a note of any that you are experiencing. This can be a great awareness and motivation tool!

The following list is to be used as an *awareness tool* for your stress level. Check off the ones you are experiencing. Keep in mind the more you check, the higher your stress level may be. If you are concerned about the number of signs and symptoms of stress you may be suffering from, this may be a great time to have a conversation with a close family member or friend, clergy or your health care professional such as doctor, and/or counselor. Whatever you choose to do, please do something proactive! Stress kills.

CHECKLIST OF SIGNS AND SYMPTOMS OF STRESS OVERLOAD

- ○ Memory Problems
- ○ Inability to concentrate
- ○ Poor judgement
- ○ Seeing only the negative
- ○ Anxious or racing thoughts
- ○ Constant worrying
- ○ Moodiness
- ○ Irritability or short temper
- ○ Agitation, inability to relax
- ○ Feeling overwhelmed
- ○ Sense of loneliness and isolation
- ○ Depression or general unhappiness
- ○ Aches and pains
- ○ Diarrhea or constipation
- ○ Nausea, dizziness
- ○ Chest pain rapid, heartbeat
- ○ Loss of sex drive
- ○ Frequent colds
- ○ Eating more or less
- ○ Sleeping too much or too little
- ○ Isolating yourself from others
- ○ Procrastinating or neglecting responsibilities
- ○ Using alcohol, cigarettes, or drugs to relax (negative coping skill)
- ○ Nervous habits (e.g. nail biting, pacing)

The Three Stages of Stress

There are three stages we go through as we encounter stressful situations over time. The phases take us through our initial stress reaction to what happens with long-term unresolved stress. These stages are called: (1) the alarm reaction, (2) resistance stage, and (3) exhaustion stage.

First, the alarm reaction. The alarm reaction is the *immediate* reaction to the stressor and consists of the initial adrenalin rush. In this stage your heart rate, blood pressure, respiratory rate, and blood sugar levels *increase* while blood flow to your digestive tract *decreases* and your immune system function *decreases*. We also know this alarm reaction as the *fight or flight* reaction and in this stage, your body is getting ready for to fight for survival or run like hell.

Second, is the *resistance stage*, also called the *adaptive stage*. When our stress levels continue to be high *and* if we do not have good healthy coping skills in place, this is the stage you will enter into next. As your stress level continues to be consistently elevated over a period of weeks, your body begins to pay a heavy price trying to keep up with the demands of the ongoing stress.

Your adrenalin and cortisol levels remain at a consistent higher than normal level and you can start experiencing the following: feelings of exasperation and impatience with trivial matters more often, and changes in your sleep quality and schedule. Your body reacts to this *high alert* mode by releasing sugars and fats into your system to compensate for the constant duress you are under. This excess of sugar and fat in your systems leads to defined changes in your physical and mental behavioral patterns.

The normal indications of this level are exhaustion, weariness, anxiousness, and forgetfulness. You may find yourself starting unhealthy coping habits such as using cigarettes, alcohol, food, and/or drugs to help you deal with your stress. You become an easy target for colds and flu as your immune response is also weakened.

The third and final stage is the exhaustion stage. If we do not find some way of easing our stress load or adopt effective self-care to cope with the ongoing stress, we can end up in a state of sheer exhaustion. As you settle into this stage, you are literally exhausted because your body can no longer keep up with the stressful demands you've placed on it. You may experience a complete loss of drive or desire to live your life. This stage symbolizes a complete breakdown of your body systems. This breakdown includes an immune system that has been almost totally eliminated. In this stage, you can experience the loss of mental equilibrium and extreme complications such as depression, panic attacks, heart disease, high blood pressure, digestive issues, and ulcers.

Take care of your body, it's the only one you will ever own!
~ Rita K. Garnto

Why Self-Care Works

OK, enough of the doom and gloom about stress. There is hope and a light at the end of the tunnel. This light has a name, and you guessed it, its name is *simple self-care*. If you recall, I talked about our autonomic nervous systems (ANS) having two parts. The first part is called fight *or flight*, and we just talked all about it and all its *lovely* attributes (read last two words with extreme sarcasm).

That brings us to the second part of the autonomic nervous system called *resting and digesting*. This will be our next area of focus. When we experience periods of calm and quiet, our resting and digesting part of our nervous systems is activated. Our bodies get to do exactly what the name suggests – our bodies have a chance to rest and heal, and digest our food properly. When this system is activated, we experience a decrease in our heart rate, blood pressure, and breathing rates. Our blood sugar levels normalize and the blood flow to our digestive tract increases. This increase blood flow allows the ingested food to be properly digested and allows for the absorption of the food's nutrients. Last, but certainly not least, our immune response strengthens. See the following for a summary of the resting and digesting response.

SUMMARY of the RESTING & DIGESTING RESPONSE:

_↓_ **Heart Rate**   _↓_ **Blood Pressure**

_↓_ **Breathing Rate**   _N_ **Blood Sugar**

_↑_ **Blood Flow to Digestive Tract**

_↑_ **Immunity**

Unplugging Helps

Earlier we talked about the so-called *forced* relaxation our ancestors experienced and how it has disappeared in our lives due to technological advances. If we are not careful and more intentional, we will end up plugged-in 24/7 without the much needed down time. Did you know that our bodies recharge and heal during your rest periods and sleep? If your rest periods become scarce or non-existent and/or your periods of sleep decrease in quality and length, what do *you* think will happen to your overall health and well-being? You know it's not going to be good and you are probably experiencing this right now.

Yes, our ancestors had an advantage over us without all that technology, but there are some simple things you can do to unwind before bedtime to allow yourself a better chance at improved quality of sleep. Here are some easy examples and if one, two, or even three of them resonate with you, make a note of them. More on making your list of self-care in the next part of the book.

- Set a time limit to turn all devices OFF approximately 30 minutes before bedtime.

- Set a bedtime and wake-up time and stick with it every day (as best as you can within 30 to 60 minutes).

- Create a night time ritual of winding down (eg. electronics off at 9:30 pm then shower and/or brush teeth, and then read a paper book, journal, meditate, or stretch right before getting into bed for sleep) AND making this ritual a habit.

- Read a paper book before turning lights out for sleep.

- Journal.

- Prepare for the next day. Plan what you are going to wear, pack your snacks/lunch.

- Create your to-do list for the next day.

- *Get it out of your head before you go to bed!* Too many things on your mind? Swirling or racing thoughts? Write them down on a piece of paper or in your journal.

- Give yourself a hug as soon as you lay down and take three deep breaths.

- Meditate, or do one or two gentle yoga poses prior to climbing into bed.

- Say a prayer of gratitude, religious prayer, or repeat a calming mantra.

Our Reality

I believe we are becoming a nation, pardon me, a **world** where anxiety and depression rule because of our consistently high stress levels AND our lack of effective and appropriate self-care. Not convinced yet? Take a look at the following statistics.

According to the World Health Organization, "Globally, 350 million people are affected by depression. If we don't act urgently, by 2030 depression will be the leading illness globally."

Mind-boggling, don't you think? Mind-boggling, don't you think? 350 million people! To make that number a little more *real* ... imagine the entire populations of the United States and Canada being affected by depression. That is a lot of people!

It amazes me, the more I open up to women about my own struggles with anxiety and depression, the more women tell me they do, too! We are killing ourselves with our stress levels, anxiety, and unrealistic expectations. Here is an excerpt from an article from Shape magazine, December 2016, regarding the increase of autoimmune diseases (remember stress decreases the ability of our immune systems to fight disease).

In fact, autoimmune diseases are increasing. "A recent review of literature concluded that worldwide rates of rheumatic, endocrinological, gastrointestinal, and neurological autoimmune diseases are increasing by 4 to 7 percent per year, with the greatest increases seen in celiac disease, type 1 diabetes, and myasthenia gravis (a rapid fatigue of the muscles), and the greatest increases occurring in countries in the Northern and Western Hemispheres," says Dr. Rutledge.

Chronic stress can not only lead to increased mental health issues and increase the incidence of autoimmune disease, but can also have a negative impact on the function of your cardiac, digestive, and endocrine systems.

I believe, the increased onset of heart disease, irritable bowel syndrome, leaky gut syndrome, diabetes, autoimmune diseases, cancer and the list goes on, is largely due to the amount of chronic stress we are under AND the lack of healthy, effective self-care strategies. The really awesome thing is that we can take a more proactive approach to our health... right now ... by taking better care of ourselves with simple self-care!

One new thing. One little thing.
That's all it takes to shift your life.

Just One Change

This brings us to the 3 steps of finding your *one* self-care key. Why start with just **one**? This isn't something I just made up one day, it was actually a message I started stumbling across awhile back. Let me explain. When I first started my private massage practice, in 2004, I came across this quote by Christina Baldwin, *When you are stuck in a spiral, to change all aspects of the spin, you need only change one thing*. At the time, like quotes can sometimes do, it struck such a chord within me I just had to tape to my bathroom mirror so I could read it every day. Over time, I began to notice how making one small change in my morning routine really did effect the outcome of my day. For example, if I did not have a good sleep and woke up with *my crabby pants on*, I told myself that it would be a great day over and over again. (Confession: the "it's going to be a great day" mantra, more often than not, would start off dripping with sarcasm and lots of eye rolling, but repeating it over and over and over and over again during the morning really did do something positive to my psyche.) Who knew?! … the day would usually end up being lighter and brighter than first expected.

Sometimes I replaced her quote with my mantra *I love and approve of myself* especially if my gremlins were on overtime beating me up mentally or if

I feel bloated or just plain icky. It worked! Gremlins quieted down. Just one change made all the difference to my day.

So, if that wasn't enough for me to really *get* the one change concept, the Universe put something else in my path to further reinforce this belief. I began reading the book, *The Power of Habit* by Charles Duhigg. In the prologue of his book, he talks about Lisa, one of the two dozen research subjects used by scientists to study people with destructive habits. Mr. Duhigg goes on to describe how by being motivated to change just one habit, which for Lisa was to quit smoking, she completely turned around her life around in less than four years. The book goes on to say, *"Over the next six months, she would replace smoking with jogging and that, in turn, changed how she ate, worked, slept, saved money, scheduled her workdays, planned for her future, and so on. She would start running half-marathons, and then a marathon, go back to school, buys a house, and get engaged"*. What an amazing transformation … starting with just one change.

Here is one more example if you left-brainers are still not quite buying it. Imagine you are flying a plane to the same old place you always fly for vacation. It's the same old, boring, stagnant place you always go, but somehow always end up there because it's a habit. Well, this time, at the beginning of your trip you point the nose of the plane just one degree off your usual course. Yes, just *one* tiny little degree. All you make is just one small change in your flight path and after flying for several hours, you are now in a completely different place! Exciting, isn't it?! Again, just one small change can make a huge world of difference.

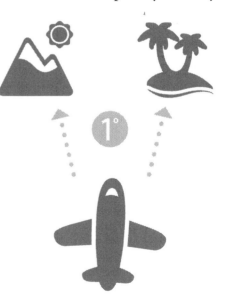

Looking at it from another angle ... you have heard of the definition of insanity, right? Insanity is defined as *doing the same thing over and over again, but expecting different results.* Been there done that. At times in my life, I just expected life to become more positive with my same, old choices and habits. Nope. Does. NOT. Work.

Let's take a look at a real life simple change. Instead of immediately jumping out of bed in the morning when your alarm goes off, you gently pull your knees to your chest and take three deep breathes. By doing this one simple stretch, your day has now started with less, and maybe even no, back discomfort or pain. Your first thought of the day can now be something positive instead of, "Oh! My back hurts!" By adding this one simple self-care, you have now created a change in your usual pattern. Perhaps that simple action slightly moves the negative thoughts to a more positive place *because* you just did something just for you! You just put **you** on the top of your priority list in that moment. That's what I call a *"Yay Me!"* moment.

With consistency, this one new thing becomes the turning point and will potentially lead to many other positive simple choices down the road. Your focus is to be consistent with this one little thing. The goal is not to overwhelm yourself because, quite honestly, most of us have enough going on in our lives and don't need to keep adding more and more stuff.

Remember: this is a PROCESS!!! This is your journey and it may take you one month to reach your goal or six months or three years, but you know what?! Somewhere in your future, you are gonna be there, my friend. How powerful is that?!

Keep It Simple Sweetie!

Step 1: The KISS Principle

Keep It Simple Sweetie. This is a much more positive spin on the old adage. Because I want this book to be about self-positivity, self-love, and self-compassion, I am using the word *sweetie* ... instead of any other "s" word.

This is the section where your brainstorming and ideas will start to flow. This is where your first step in your simple self-care journey starts to take shape. I'm excited for you! When was the last time you heard these words ... this is all about *you*? Probably not lately, or even often enough.

But as much as your friend, "Veronica", loves to run and get her mental, emotional, physical, and spiritual self-care from running, it does not have to be your thing and may, absolutely *not* be your thing. And that, my friend, is *absolutely perfect*. This journey isn't about "Veronica", it's about you! Once in a while you need to stop, regroup, get grounded, and listen to your inner self. Ask yourself, "What do *I* like to do?"

I feel too often we get lost in everyone else's life and their choices and forget about what matters to us. Single. Married. No children. You can still can lost in your career, business, or someone else's drama. This book and my thought process is focused on what resonates with you. What makes **you** want to take better care of yourself? What makes **you** feel better about yourself? What lowers **your** stress level and what is going to help **you** get to where **you** want to go in **your** life, health, and well-being?

I do not care what your friend A or B does for self-care because I care about you (unless, of course, she is reading this book and then she would be you.)

Why do I make such a big deal of this process being *all about you*?

Because this is your journey and no one else's, and we are all created differently with our own quirks, nuances, subtle, and obvious differences. This simple self-care journey belongs to you and only you. Focusing on your needs, allows a greater sense of self-awareness which, I think, is really important in order to reach your goals.

Can you get ideas, help, and support from others?
Absolutely!

Can you bitch and vent and stomp your feet and share your frustrations and triumphs with others?
Please do! Get as much support from others as possible.

Your List

On to your list of self-care preferences. Before we start, let's go over the definition of self-care again so you have a clear idea of what kinds of things to write down on your list.

SELF-CARE is *any intentional action you take to care for your mental, emotional, physical, and spiritual health.*

Grab a writing utensil and blank piece of paper or better yet, a journal or notebook. If you prefer to work on your laptop, please do so. I am of the pencil and paper generation and I love to brainstorm with a pen in my hand writing on paper. When I journal, I will often pick different colors to write with depending on my mood. There is just something about the tactile feel of the paper and pen that helps clear my mind.

To start this brainstorming process, begin listing all the self-care things that you would like to do or maybe have never done, but would like to try. The point of this exercise is just to free-write and look inside yourself to really become aware of what you can and will do for self-care.

The DO's:

1. Make this about YOU!
2. Throw away any preconceived notions and unrealistic expectations.
3. Pick self-care that you are *financially, mentally, emotionally, spiritually, mentally,* and *physically* able to do.
   (This is very important. By understanding *your* constraints and limitations, you will be setting yourself up for success. By creating

a list of doable self-care choices, you're allowing yourself to accomplish this goal easily.)

The do NOT's:

1. Do NOT allow anyone else's expectations to dictate this list.
2. Do NOT use the words … *should, could, have to.*
3. Do NOT limit yourself.

Here is a list of questions to help you if you are stuck or your brain needs a little shove in the right direction. Please do not answer every question. Some of the questions may seem a little redundant, but I have tried to frame them in different ways. Because we all learn via different pathways, some questions may be easier for you to answer than others. Pick the ones that resonate the most with you. It *is* all about you!

1. What activities makes me feel good mentally? Happy?

_____

_____

_____

2. What activities make me feel good about myself?

_____

_____

_____

3. How do I "get out of my head"?

_____

_____

_____

4. What activities help clear my head and think more clearly?

_____

_____

_____

5. What activities help calm me down?

_____

_____

_____

6. What activities decrease my stress level?

_____

_____

_____

7. What do I like to do to help recharge my energy level after a long, tiring day?

_____

_____

_____

8. What helps me diffuse my temper?

_____

_____

_____

9. How do I gain clarity in my thoughts?

_____

_____

_____

10. What helps me slow down and appreciate life?

_____

_____

_____

11. What helps me feel empowered?

_____

_____

_____

12. What helps me feel like I have some control in my life?

_____

_____

_____

13. What gives me peace?

_____

_____

_____

14. What brings peace to my often chaotic and stressful day?

_____

_____

_____

15. What helps me slow down?

_____

_____

_____

16. What helps me become more mindful/more in the present?

_____

_____

_____

17. What helps me appreciate me for me?

_____

_____

_____

18. What physical activity helps boost my emotional, mental, and/or spiritual self?

_____

_____

_____

19. My favorite inspirational quote is:

_____

_____

_____

20. My favorite mantra is:

_____

_____

_____

21. My favorite scripture is:

_____

_____

_____

22. What is written on my mirror to inspire me?

_____

_____

_____

23. How does deep breathing help calm me/decrease my stress level?

_____

_____

_____

24. What helps me pick myself up emotionally? Mentally? Spiritually?

_____

_____

_____

25. Do I prefer walking or other moving activity over journaling to reduce my stress level or calm down?

_____

_____

_____

26. Do I prefer journaling or meditating over walking to reduce my stress level or calm down?

_____

_____

_____

27. What feeds my soul?

_____

_____

_____

28. What feeds my spirit?

_____

_____

_____

29. What activities recharge me?

_____

_____

_____

30. What activities fill my emotional bank account?

_____

_____

_____

31. What am I not doing now that I would like to start doing that would make a difference in my well-being?

_____

_____

_____

On the following page, I have created a table with some of many self-care choices out there. This table is full of examples of all different kinds of self-care. I'm sure you would be able to add to the list and please feel free to add others on the bottom of the list or anywhere on the page. (I would love to hear about your self-care so please feel free to send me an email.) The beauty of having all these options in one place is that this can become your self-care resource list down the road.

Back to the list ... I am honestly not trying to stress you out with all the choices! I am merely hoping to make you be aware of how many choices and options you really have.

Keep in mind that this is just an overview of self-care and I will be walking you through every step with more detail in the following sections. Please do not get caught up in the overwhelm of this large list. Just observe the list and make note of what jumps out at you.

Examples of Self-Care:

a nap	one glass of wine	being outside
aromatherapy	work on good posture	coloring
attending Taekwondo Class	knitting/needlework	join small church group
deep breathing	running	walking
drink a smoothie	drink lots of water	drink water with lemon
drumming	warm cup of tea	Epsom salt bath
floss daily	walk with a buddy	7-9 hours of sleep
hiking	walking your dog	listening to soothing music
lifting weights	biking	cycling class
mantras	nutritional eating	10 min quiet time
massage	chiropractic	yoga
pedicure	facials	manicure
Pilates	bubble bath	stretching
practice taekwondo	talk with a friend/sister	10 squats daily
reading fiction	reading scripture	journaling
singing	meditating	chanting
sunshine	dancing	playing with the kids
supplements	motivational quotes	positive affirmations
tai chi	joining a book club	line dancing
attend church regularly	counseling	drink green juice

Now it is your turn to create your list.
On your mark.
Get set.
Write!

Simple Self-Care is any intentional self-care action that is easy, not rocket-science nor complex, and effortlessly slides into your day.

Simple Self-Care

Now, you have your general list of self-care options. Keep in mind this is the first of three steps to finding your *one new thing*. The self-care options you have written down are the ones that you *can* do, and appeal to you. Most likely some of these self-care choices, if not most of them, may take some kind of time commitment. This has been one of the problems ... you feel you don't have the time to do self-care because you are too busy, too tired, or too overwhelmed. Again, this book is about finding the simple things that you can *slide effortlessly* into your day without the added stress and anxiety of trying to find time to squeeze one more thing into your already hectic schedule.

This section of the book is all about giving you examples of *simple* self-care. Simple self-care is the kind of self-care that will effortlessly slide into your day. As you read through this next part, please keep your self-care list from the previous section close-by to make note of any of the simple self-care moves that appeal to you. Remember: this is all about *you*!

A quick review: The definition of self-care is any intentional action you take to care for your mental, emotional, physical, and spiritual health. Simple self-care is any intentional self-care action that is *easy, not rocket-science nor complex, and effortlessly slides into your day*.

For this next section, I welcome you to join Ms. Sophie Self-Care on her simple self-care journey demonstrating many simple self-care choices. This following section is a compilation of tips, hints, and suggestions I have learned from many different sources in my journey. It is by no means a complete list and I would love to hear from you about your simple self-care. Let's grow this section together!

As you go through the following choices please do not go into overwhelm. If you like any or all of these moves, write them on your list. Rest assured, we will be narrowing all your choices down to just one simple self-care choice effortlessly. As time goes on and your journey continues, you will be adding one more simple self-care at a time, but not until you are ready to do so. More on that later.

1. Give-Yourself-a-Hug

Before getting out of bed in the morning, slowly bring your knees towards your chest and hold. Take a few slow, deep breaths. This is also great to do at bedtime or anytime, for that matter, as long as you are able to lay down comfortably in a safe place. This move helps ease the tension out of the lower back at any time during the day.

Tip: this is your time so make it all about you!

The Why:

Stretching relaxes your mind, tunes up your body, and makes you feel great. Stretching our lower backs daily is also very important. According to the American Chiropractic Association, here are a few interesting facts about back pain:

- Low back pain is the single leading cause of disability worldwide, according to the Global Burden of Disease 2010.
- Back pain is one of the most common reasons for missed work. In fact, back pain is the second most common reason for visits to the doctor's office, outnumbered only by upper-respiratory infections.
- One-half of all working Americans admit to having back pain symptoms each year.
- Experts estimate that as much as 80% of the population will experience a back problem at some time in their lives.
- Most cases of back pain are mechanical or non-organic—meaning they are not caused by serious conditions, such as inflammatory arthritis, infection, fracture or cancer.

- Americans spend at least $50 billion each year on back pain—and that's just for the more easily identified costs.

Most stretched muscles: gluteus maximus, and muscles along the spine and lower back.

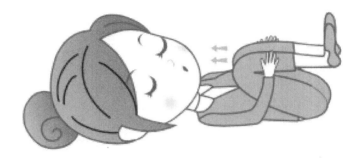

This movement can also be done with one knee at a time for a deeper stretch in the back & glutes along with hamstrings of the straight leg.

Muscles stretched in straight leg include hamstrings, and gluteus medius.

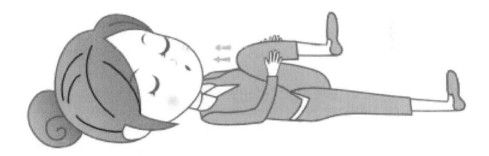

Added Tip: bringing your knee towards your armpit or opposite shoulder instead of your chest, will increase the stretch in the muscles listed above.

2. Getting out of Bed the *Right* Way

Yes, there is a right way and a *wrong* way of getting out of bed. Sitting up by thrusting your head forward and jerking your body to an upright position, can aggravate already tight back and neck muscles. Some days it is tough enough getting out of bed without the added aches and pains.

Next, Sophie shows you two of the steps to getting out of bed the right way to lessen back and neck strain. Combining the morning hug with this move, is a sure way to help your back and you feel better and more able to begin your day with a positive start and more importantly, less pain.

First, roll over onto your side facing the side of the bed you wish to get up on. Secondly, as you gently push yourself up into a seated position using your arms, hang your legs off the side of the bed. When you are in a complete sitting position, pause for a moment, and make sure your feet are flat on the floor before you push yourself up to a standing position.

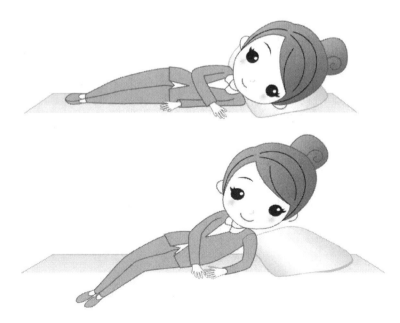

The Why:

To prevent straining your lower back and neck when getting up. If you already have issues in these areas, this simple self-care tip can prevent any further aggravation, discomfort, and pain. This move can also be used for getting up from the couch, and floor.

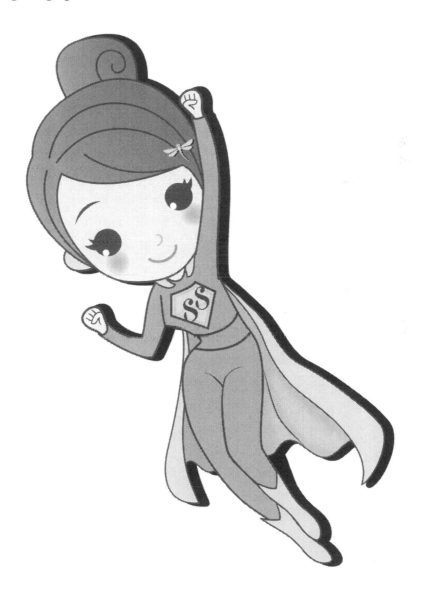

3. Reach UP

Reaching up can be done just about anywhere and anytime. The purpose is to move your body in a way that it does not normally move during the day – unless of course, you stack things on high shelves all day as your job.

If you think about it, what position are we in most often during the day while working on the computer, doing household chores, and driving? We are typically in what is called, an anteriorly rotated position (shoulders rounded forward). So, what better way to counteract that forward rotation then to reach up and stretch towards the sky.

The Why:

Stretching relaxes your mind, tunes up your body, and makes you feel great. There exists a neuromuscular law called **DAVIS' LAW** and it is one of the many neuromuscular laws governing the relationship between the nerves and muscles. Like the Law of Gravity, Davis' Law is a known fact and is a law of nature.

Davis' Law states that *when the two muscle ends become closer together, the strength of the muscle increases.* In other words, when a muscle becomes shorter, it becomes stronger and when a muscle becomes stronger it becomes shorter. The opposite is also true. When a muscle becomes longer (or stretched), it becomes weaker.

A practical example would be the chest muscles. The more we slouch and lean forward during our daily activities, the shorter our chest muscles get. According to Davis' law, as our chest muscles shorten, they are also getting stronger and thereby increasing the forward pull of our shoulders. Now think about what is happening to your upper and mid back muscles. The muscles of the upper and mid back have the opposite action to the chest muscles and we use them to maintain good upright posture. When we chronically slouch forward, the upper back muscles are being stretched forward thereby getting longer, and weaker. And yet, they continue to work overtime trying to counteract the forward pull of the chest muscles by pulling backward. (Note: there many more muscle groups involved in this process. I have only mentioned the chest and back muscles to keep the concept as simple as possible.)

Ever notice a burning sensation or dull ache in between your shoulder blades? This is a signal that your back muscles are working overtime, getting tired, and are not getting enough oxygen. This feeling is just like *muscle burn* you experience when exerting your body during exercise. This burning sensation is caused by the build-up of lactic acid due to lack of oxygen in the muscles.

Most stretched muscles: chest, shoulder, and bicep muscles.

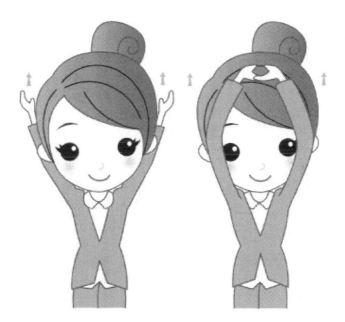

4. Reach OUT

As with all these movements, you should move slowly and gently into these positions. This is about movement and increasing blood flow to tight muscles and not about making major gains in your flexibility or becoming a contortionist.

Place your feet shoulder width apart or slightly wider depending on your comfort and balance. Lift your arms out to your sides, keeping your arms straight, up to shoulder height to form a "T". Pause. Take a deep breath. Gently squeeze your shoulder blades together and relax your upper trapezius muscles so you are not scrunching your shoulders up to your ears. Rotate your hands so your thumbs are pointing up to the ceiling. Feel the gentle stretch in your chest. For a little more stretch, while keeping your arms straight and shoulders down, move your thumbs towards the back of the room.

The Why:

As with the Reach Up movement, reaching out will stretch and loosen tight chest and shoulder muscles. When muscles become less tense and tight, more blood flow is able to reach the muscles and this translates into delivery of more oxygen and food to help calm tight, hurting muscles. As you loosen tight chest muscles, you are easing the strain and pull on your upper back muscles.

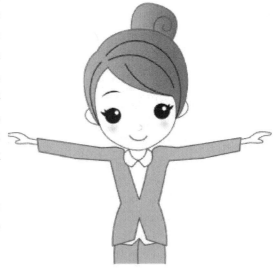

Most stretched muscles: chest, shoulder, and bicep muscles.

5. Chest Stretch on Exercise Ball

This simple self-care movement takes the last chest stretch and takes it a step further. By using an exercise ball and gravity, you will be able to get even more of a stretch throughout your chest area. I like to do this one at the end of day by just relaxing in the position described below for a couple of minutes. It is amazing how much your aching back muscles will appreciate this move.

You will need an appropriately sized exercise ball for this movement. The appropriate size can typically be found on the outside of the box or package the ball comes in and is based on your height. Below are recommendations found on https://www.spine-health.com/wellness/exercise/choosing-right-exercise-ball

Choosing the Right Exercise Ball

Exercise ball diameter	Person's height
55 cm	5'1"– 5'8"
65 cm	5'9"– 6'2"
75 cm	6'3"– 6'7"
85 cm	6'8" and taller

A few comments about the stability ball. It can provide a great opportunity for stretching, but using the ball does require balance and falling or sliding off the ball onto the floor with possible injury can occur. Keeping your feet anchored on the floor and having the right size ball will help greatly with your balance. When you are using the ball, make sure you have a sufficient open floor space around you to minimize the danger of rolling into or falling onto objects that may inflict pain. If you are overweight, older, or maybe just out of shape, you may find it easier to balance on a larger, slightly less-inflated ball. These particular recommendations come from the American Council on Exercise. As with any new exercise, please consult your health care professional with any concerns you have prior to starting.

Sit on the ball with feet slightly apart so you are comfortable and can maintain good balance and posture. Slowly walk your feet away from the ball as you slowly place your upper body onto the ball. You are in correct position when your head comes to rest on the ball and feels supported. See Sophie below.

Note: make sure your head and neck are well supported by the ball to prevent strain of your neck muscles.

Most stretched muscles: chest, shoulder, and bicep muscles.

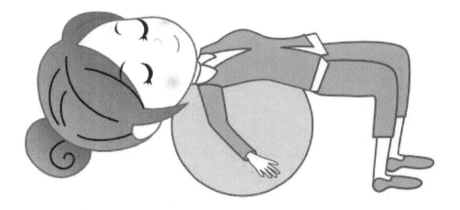

6. Let's Twist

Stand upright with feet hip width apart, knees slightly bent, and arms extended straight out from your sides. Take a deep breath in and as you exhale, slowly rotate to the left looking over your left shoulder and keeping your arms extended and straight.

Note to self: Watch out for walls, people, and other obstacles nearby!

Inhale as you return to the center. Now, slowly rotate to the right as you exhale looking over your right shoulder and repeat the movement several times. Gentle and slow movements.

The Why:

The gentle twisting movement helps keep your tiny spinal muscles (the multifidi, rotatores, interspinales, and intertransversarii) between your vertebrae moving and flexible. You are also engaging your internal and external obliques (your abdominal muscles on your sides) as well as chest, shoulder, and lower back muscles.

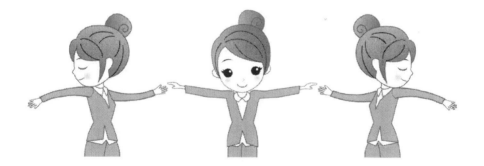

7. Stretching while brushing your teeth

I like to make use of my teeth brushing time to stretch. It's simple, easy, and doesn't take away time from my day. We are supposed to be brushing for 2 minutes, right, so why not multitask just a little?

To do this stretch, stand back from the counter a foot or two (this distance will vary depending on your leg length and flexibility). Then simply place one foot on the edge of the bathroom counter. If the counter edge is too high or if this position is uncomfortable, place your foot on the edge of the bathtub or toilet. (Note to self: close toilet lid first just in case of foot slippage.)

Keeping your upper body **upright** (NO bending forward at the hips), gently push your hips forward. You should feel this stretch in your straight leg near or at the place where your leg attaches to our body. As with all stretching, there should be NO pain. A slight pulling or discomfort in this area is normal and expected. Relax your shoulders and breathe … yes, all while brushing your teeth.

The Why:

Often, the reason our lower backs hurt is because our hip flexors are too tight. Hip flexors are the muscles that help us bend forward and consist of our quadriceps, iliopsoas muscles, and to a lesser extent sartorius. From all the sitting we do, these muscles in the front of our bodies become overworked and tight. (Remember Davis' Law?) This tightening can cause our pelvis to be pulled forward creating an imbalance with stretching and weakening of our lower back muscles. Reducing this imbalance by loosening our hip flexors, can help ease the strain and pain in our lower backs.

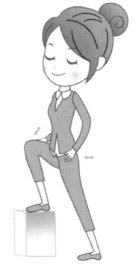

Most Stretched Muscles: quadriceps and iliopsoas muscles.

8. Shoulder scrunches

What better way to relieve tension in your shoulders then with easy, simple shoulder shrugs?

As you take a deep breath in, pull and scrunch your shoulders up to your ears ...hold, hold. As you exhale, let them drop and relax. Repeat. And repeat again. This is so easy and simple to do that you can slide it into your day just about anytime, anywhere.

The Why:

Earlier, I mentioned that tight muscles can a have decreased blood flow and this is not a good thing. Our muscles need good blood flow to remain healthy, functioning, and pain-free. Blood flow distributes oxygen and nutrients throughout our bodies, muscles included, and removes the toxic waste products of metabolism.

Imagine all the tiny blood vessels feeding your muscles are like the garden hoses that you use to water your outside plants. When you kink the hose, less water flows through the hose. This is a similar concept with the blood vessels in your muscles. When your muscles are tight, they squeeze and "kink" the blood vessels so they are unable to deliver optimal blood flow, oxygen, and nutrients to the muscles and are unable to effectively remove the toxic waste products. These toxic waste products – lactic acid, bradykinin - can trigger discomfort and pain. Think of that *burning* sensation you feel in your legs during an intense workout or between your shoulder blades when sitting in front of the computer for long periods of time – that is caused by a buildup of lactic acid from the muscles not getting enough oxygen.

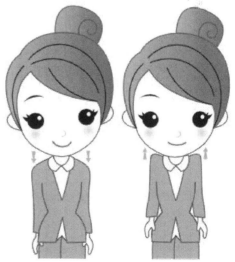

Movement, including the contraction and relaxation sequence, helps the muscles relax overall and thereby, allows for more efficient blood flow, more oxygen, and more nutrients being delivered to the muscles. This increased blood flow can also decrease this burning sensation as the toxic waste products are flushed away. I have, perhaps, over-simplified this process in hopes to give you a clearer picture of what is going on in those poor, overused, tired muscles of yours.

Muscles Used: upper trapezius, levator scapulae (their action is to elevate your shoulder blades)

9. A Few More Steps

I have been wearing a pedometer for several years now. I am hesitant to mention the brand as I do not want to appear that I am endorsing any particular company. There are a lot of good ones out there.

What's great about wearing a pedometer is that you really get to see how many steps you take during the day. For me, it has acted as a motivator to be a little more active especially if you set a daily goal such as 5,000 steps or maybe even 8,000 or 10,000 steps.

I have been known to walk circles around the kitchen, dining room, and all over the house right before I go to bed to get my steps in and meet my goal. A girl has got to do what a girl has got to do! A *Yay Me!* moment, indeed.

The Why:

Based loosely on my calculations using my pedometer, if I were to take an extra 100 steps per day, in one year I will have walked an extra 18 miles! Wow! Now 100 steps are really not very much if you think about it AND here are some simple suggestions to get those extra steps.

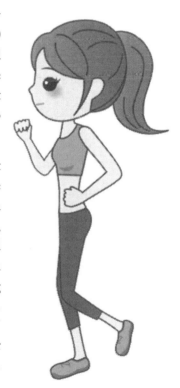

At home or the office, walk to the furthest bathroom when you need to go. At the office, that may mean walking up or down a flight of stairs ... even better! At home, for example, my office is on the second floor and I have my daughters' bathroom right next door to me. I am now walking downstairs to the master bathroom to go. Think of all those extra steps especially if I drink way too much water, tea, and/or coffee. Go Mom! ... oops, pardon the pun.

Another idea is to park a little further away from your office door when going to work or at the store when running errands. How about taking the stairs instead of the elevator? Too many flights of stairs? How about taking the stairs part of the way? Be creative. Think outside of the box. Those steps will add up!

Crazy as this may sound, you can also step in place or step side to side when waiting for the microwave or coffee or tea to brew. Add a twist when touching elbows to knees for added benefit. *Get moving ladies with a few more steps!* It's simple, easy, and not rocket science.

10. Deep Breathing

What better way to relieve tension in your whole body, including your mind and spirit, than with a pause and some deep breaths?

Step 1: Pause and stop what you are doing ... where and when it is SAFE, of course.

Step 2: Get comfortable. If you are sitting, place feet flat on the floor and hands held loosely in your lap. If you are standing, place your feet a comfortable width apart to maintain good balance and let your arms hang loosely at your sides.

Step 3: As you breathe in, allow your lower abdomen to expand outward.

Step 4: As you exhale, contract your abdomen slightly so it moves inward.

Step 5: Repeat 3 to 6 times or until you feel your stress level decrease.

This is so easy and simple to do that you can slide it into your day just about anytime, anywhere ... of course, as long as you are not operating any heavy machinery or doing something that requires your attention!

The Why:

I find it amazing how this very simple deep breathing exercise will activate the part of your nervous system, the parasympathetic nervous system, that controls the *resting and digesting* impulses in your body. Remember we talked about your nervous system and how it functions during both calm and stressful time. By simply pausing and taking some deep breaths, you can lower your heart rate, blood pressure, breathing rate, along with increasing the blood flow to your digestive tract (thereby allowing your body to use the nutrients you have consumed). Ommmmm ....

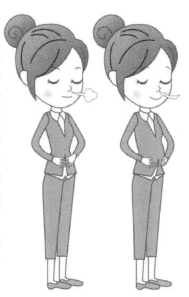

11. Pause. Be Still.

Being still. Do you even remember what that is? Today in our fast-paced world it seems we expect ourselves to always be doing something and on the go. It is amazing how pausing for just a moment or two and just *being still* can be great for bringing down stress levels. Add in a few deep breaths and you have got an amazingly simple way to recover after a stressful encounter, client phone call, tantrum, or prepare for an upcoming stressful situation. Being still can be done sitting up or lying down. Just make sure you are in a safe place and do not risk any injury to yourself.

The Why:

When we are on the hectic go and in the *fight or flight* mode – discussed in an earlier part of the book - one of the things that stops working is our cognitive thinking. According to dictionary.com, cognitive thinking is defined as relating to the mental processes of perception, memory, judgement and reasoning. In other words, cognitive thinking involves higher level thinking and decision making. When we stop using our cognitive thinking, we are less able and less likely to make good decisions because when we are in survival mode, we rely more on our primitive instincts to guide us. This can lead to spur of the moment decisions that are not always in our best interest.

As described in the book ***The Charisma Myth*** by **Olivia Fox Cabane**,

> *"Have you ever become paralyzed in the middle of an exam or had the experience of stage fright? Like a deer in headlights, you freeze, your heart races, your palms get sweaty. You're desperately trying to remember what you'd planned to say or do, but your mind is blank. Your higher cognitive functions, have shut down."*

In the moment of a crisis or even a perceived crisis, is a good time to be still and collect our thoughts. This will let our bodies restore some important mental functions as well as physical ones.

12. Being Mindful

Being mindful is very similar to being still. Being mindful is more intentional of being aware of your immediate surroundings. Being in the moment. Being aware of what your body is feeling and what messages you have running in your head right at this moment. Today in this fast-paced world, it seems, we are either thinking about our to-do lists, what *needs* to be done (future), or what we *should* have done (past). It is amazing how being mindful for just a minute or two can help us become more aware of this very moment, be present in the now, and slow down just a little.

Being mindful can be done anywhere. Just look around you and start noticing the details of your environment. What sounds can you hear? What colors stand out the most? If you are outside, make note of the color of the sky, the number of clouds, the trees, the flowers ... you get idea. Use your five senses and connect with each one.

Not quite working for you? ... wiggle your toes. Yes, wiggle your toes. Take your shoes off and feel the ground with your feet. Ask yourself ... is the surface beneath my feet soft, hard, cold, or warm? Is this feeling comfortable? Stretch your toes. Curl your toes. How do your feet feel? Are they cramped, tired, hot, puffy, or perfect?

This is a great exercise for bringing you back to the present and out of the past or future. If you are in a conversation and you find your mind wandering or maybe you are not fully engaged, wiggle our toes to bring you back to the present.

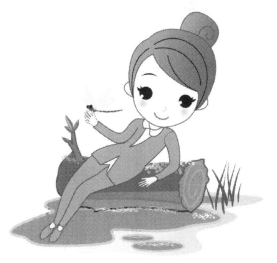

Life is too short and if we are not living in the now, life

will just slip away. I don't know about you, but I don't want to wake up one morning and realize that I am 80 years old wondering, "Where did my life go?"

The Why:

Being more present can help reduce stress and anxiety by allowing your brain to focus on what is happening right now. Rather than **over** estimating what *might be* and being stuck in the future, we can focus on *what is* in the here and now. Rather than focusing on what we *should* have said, done, thought (which really is a waste of energy as the past can't be changed), just be here and now. Here and now is where the change and magic happens!

13. Ragdoll

This has to be one of my all-time favorite poses! I use it to ease lower back tightness, achiness, and to ease neck and shoulder tension. Keeping your legs are straight, this stretch can also be used to stretch the calves and hamstrings. When I first started doing it, my hands would hang down around my knee level. Now, I can put my hands flat on the floor with my elbows bent. Yes, it took me several years of consistently doing this pose for me to achieve those results. My flexibility is better now than it was when I was 25! Consistency really does pay off!

Step 1: Stand with your feet hip width apart, toes pointing forward. *(Note:* If you are familiar with this pose and would like to add more stretch for your hips, turn your feet in slightly.)

Step 2: Bring your hands to your hips, bend your knees slightly.

Step 3: Imagine your hips are a hinge as you bend forward with a flat back as far as you comfortably can bend.

Note: If you have lower back issues, go to next stretch. Depending on the severity of your back issues, you may want to talk to your physician first, before doing this pose. Always proceed slowly and walk your hands down to your knees to support your upper body. If at any time you experience any discomfort, please slowly return to standing and do not attempt this pose until:

a. you have been cleared by your doctor or other healthcare professional,

b. you have increased the flexibility of your back using some of the other gentle back poses,

c. you no longer experience any back discomfort and/or pain as you move into this pose, or

d. decide you don't like this pose and it is not for you!

Step 4: Cross your arms and hold onto opposite elbows and allow your upper body to hang like a *ragdoll*.

Step 5: Stay in the pose for 3 to 6 deep breaths, breathing in and out through your nose.

Step 6: To come out of the pose, bring your hands to your hips keeping your knees slightly bent. On inhalation, gently roll your back, one vertebrae at a time, to a standing position.

The Why:

Stretching relaxes your mind, tunes up your body, and makes you feel great. Putting those overused muscles in a different position, can allow them to relax and allow for increased blood flow. Instant pain relief!

Muscles Most Stretched: upper and lower back, neck, hamstrings, and calves

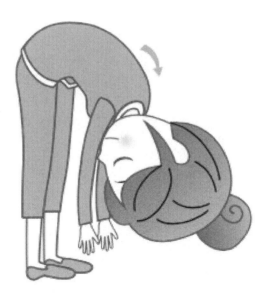

14. Seated Lower Back Stretch

If the ragdoll stretch causes any discomfort and/or pain, use this one instead. In this movement, your lower back is supported by placing your chest on your upper legs, thereby, reducing the strain on your lower back.

Sit upright in a chair with your feet and legs apart. Take a deep breath in and as you slowly exhale, slowly lean forward rounding your upper back. Continue to bend at the waist as you exhale until your head and abdomen are as low as they can go. Allow your upper body rest on your legs and allow your head to hang down loosely. (Not to be done after ingesting a large meal!)

The Why:

Stretching relaxes your mind, tunes up your body, and makes you feel great. Putting those overused muscles in a different position, can allow them to relax and allow for increased blood flow. Instant pain relief!

Most stretched muscles: back and neck

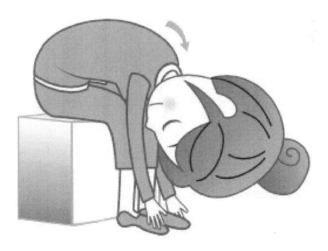

15. Ice, Baby, Ice

Because of all my joint issues, knees especially, ice has become my best friend at times. After a long taekwondo class, walk, or just a bad day, I ice my knees. On days that my shoulders or back hurt, I use ice as one of my first go-to's to reduce the swelling, inflammation, and discomfort.

Word of caution: ice may or may not work for you depending on your type of issue. It is a matter of seeing your healthcare professional and trying it out. Sometimes I will use ice on particularly painful area of my body and it does **not** feel better. I may then try moist heat instead. If you have chronically tight neck, shoulder, and or back muscles, moist heat may be a better choice for you and see #16 for more info on that. A good rule of thumb: if the injury has happened within the last 72 hours, use ice. This, again, is only a guideline and it often takes trial and error to see what works best for you.

I have also used ice and heat. If you decide to try this method of alternating ice and heat, always start with ice and end with ice. For example, ice the area for a few minutes then apply moist heat for a few minutes, repeat with the ice and heat and then end with ice.

Applying ice has a time limit! **Do not** *over ice* **as this can impede your body's healing process**.

There are a variety of ways to use ice. It can be as simple and inexpensive as buying a frozen bag of veggies (peas, or corn work great) on sale and using that as your ice pack. (Note: make sure to clearly mark this bag for "icing only" so not to confuse it for a meal item.)

This little bag of frozen veggies is great for tucking into the back of your pants for lower back issues or under the strap of your bra for shoulder pain. Using the ice pack in this way, allows you to continue to be mobile and do what you need to do and not have to sit in one place for 10 to 20 minutes. I also believe that having movement in the affected area while icing is beneficial to the whole process. I do not have research to back this up, but it has worked well for me. Be careful not to leave the ice on for too long (no longer than 20 minutes) as this can potentially impede the healing process if blood flow is reduced for too long of a period.

For icing my knees, I have invested in knee wraps. These ice packs have two straps with Velcro and I can wrap them around my knees and continue to be mobile or sit with my legs elevated. For more info on the ice wraps I use, please see the resource section.

For more severe swelling, you can also do ice *massage*. This is a little more labor intensive and messy, but is great when you are experiencing a particularly bad injury/swelling issue. This ice massage requires ice frozen in a cup and a towel or two. The great thing about ice massage is that it takes a maximum of five minutes so it's quick, but keep in mind it takes more attention to detail as you can give yourself frostbite if not done correctly. (Yup, been there done that! Ouch!) For more information on ice massage, please also turn to the resource section.

Bonus: A great little tip I learned from my physical therapist ... after a workout when waiting for the shower to warm up, put your injured, swollen, or aching joint under the stream of cold water. Yes, not very pleasant and takes a little ... ok, a lot ... of determination at times especially in the winter, but I find that it helps reduce the *heat* (inflammation) in my knees and makes them feel better instantly. Quick, easy, and simple.

The Why:

Ice is great at reducing swelling and inflammation by reducing blood flow to the injured area. It is also great at providing temporary pain relief after an acute or traumatic injury. What I learned in massage school is the healing properties of icing also include the warming up process of the injured area *after* the ice is removed. Let me explain. When you ice your knee for example, you are reducing the blood flow to that area because the ice is causing the blood vessels to constrict and reducing the swelling and inflammation. When the ice is removed and the area slowly warms up, the blood flow increases to the area bringing with it food, oxygen, and other healing components. This can potentially speed up the healing process. I know, for me, the ice helps greatly at reducing the chronic swelling in my knees. Remember that I have been diagnosed with osteoarthritis by a physician and have worked extensively with my physical therapist over the years so if you have any questions, please ask your health care professional.

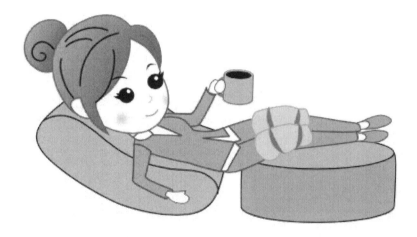

16. Moist Heat

I feel that moist heat penetrates the muscles better than dry heat. Standing still for a few minutes in the stream of hot water while you shower can do wonders for tight shoulder and back muscles. (A warm bath ... even "awesomer"!) The key words are *standing still*. Savor your time alone even if it is just for a few minutes. Take a few deep breaths. Feel the water hitting your back and running down to your feet (mindfulness). Adding a few simple shoulder rolls or the ragdoll pose (careful not to get water up your nose!) increases the benefit of the heat.

Wake up with a headache or tight shoulder (upper trapezius) muscles. Not convenient to take a shower or it's the middle of the day? Grab a flaxseed neck wrap, pop it in the microwave, and place it on your shoulders. Ahhhhhh ...! Between the heat and the weight of the neck wrap, you can literally feel your shoulders relax. Lower back tightness ... tuck the heated flaxseed wrap in your pants or behind you when you are sitting or lying down.

The Why:

Heat increases blood flow to the muscles. This increase in blood flow brings much needed oxygen and food to the muscles and flushes out toxic waste products. This entire process helps tight muscles relax and stop hurting. Moist heat is great for chronically tight muscles.

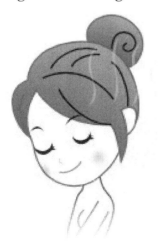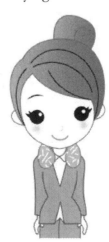

17. Tennis Ball "Therapy"

Sometimes we just have a pain in the tush or between the shoulder blades that just won't go away with simple movement or stretching. This is where tennis ball therapy comes in.

I find *tennis ball therapy* very effective. It is a fixture in my self-care arsenal and have recommended it to many of my massage clients over the years as well. It is simple to do and inexpensive.

Simply take the tennis ball and place it underneath the area of discomfort while lying on the floor. For example, if you have been sitting for long periods of time in front of the computer and you have a burning ache between your shoulder blades. While lying down on the floor, place the tennis ball directly under the area of discomfort between your shoulder blades. You may have to make some minor adjustments to the position of the tennis ball to get just the right spot. Lean into the tennis ball as much as the pain/discomfort will allow and breathe. Do not roll around on the tennis ball. Do NOT place it under bone … OUCH!! Place the tennis ball under soft tissue only.

This technique is more about acupressure and releasing the tight muscles with a steady pressure rather than a lot of movement. Hope that makes sense. This therapy is also great for hips, glutes, feet, and wherever else you may find it effective.

TIP: If you are undertaking a long road trip in the car, take a tennis ball along and place it under different areas of your glutes and even your low back to help ease the tension of long periods of sitting.

Word of Caution: if you have a dog, especially any kind of lab or retriever mix, make sure he/she does not see you place the ball underneath you as your dog may try to create an interesting game of hide and seek with you and the ball. Fun, but not necessarily effective while using this simple self-care technique.

The Why:

The shape and size of the tennis ball along with your body weight is great for targeting trigger points in your tight muscles. What is a *trigger point?* A trigger point is a hyper-irritable spot located within a taut band of muscle which often refers pain to other parts of the body when touched or compressed. These trigger points are usually caused by muscle overload (overuse of that individual muscle or muscle group), an injury, or stress. Trigger point therapy consists of the application of constant pressure to the trigger point to help it release and thereby decreasing its painful effects and dysfunction in other parts of the body.

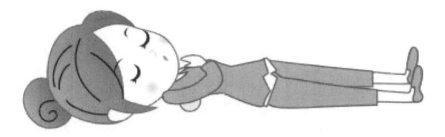

Tennis ball therapy … easy, peasy, lemon squeezy.

At one time or another, I have used all of these simple self-care techniques. All the suggestions in the book have been tried and tested by me. You may find that one of the listed simple self-care moves inspires you to create a new version that works better for you. I would love to hear about what works best for you. If any of these simple self-care moves resonate with you, add them to your self-care list.

> # *You have to listen to what resonates within your own gut. You find your direction there. Your voice comes out.*
>
> ## *~ Kathy Mattea*

Step 2: It Must Resonate

Each of us are unique thinkers and we are unique in the way we do things. One size does *not* fit all. This step is about finding what works for you in your life story. After all, this is what this book is all about … finding what works for you, my friend.

Our goal in this chapter is to narrow down on your list of self-care by:

a. finding the self-care that *resonates* with you and

b. *fits* into your life story.

Remember, all life stories are unique and deserve to be celebrated. I believe, that by you making these choices at this particular moment in time, you are setting yourself up for success. Why? Because you are picking the one change you are going to start with. Someone didn't tell you what to do or when to do it. You get to decide that and in doing so, you are empowering yourself. You are taking a little piece of control back by being ready to make the decision to start your one new thing.

By deciding what is going to work for you, you are taking on more responsibility for your needs. This requires you to have an increased self-awareness and maybe even an increased honesty and openness with yourself. This may be a little intimidating or feel strange if you are not used to being self-aware. This feeling that you are taking back some control, I am hoping will lift your spirit and help you closer towards believing and achieving. I call this the *"Yes, I can with ease"* attitude. It's all about the small steps. It's about the little battles that we win with ourselves every day that add up to the bigger victories and the bigger successes that we will accomplish.

Enter the verb … **to resonate.** According to dictionary.com, the word origin of to *resonate* is from the Latin *resonāre* and is a verb meaning to *produce a positive feeling, emotional response, or opinion.*

I like to think that when something resonates with me, it just *feels right.* It feels like it was meant for me and it greatly appeals to me. My solar plexus gives me a signal that it is the right choice for me. For example, when I go to a new restaurant and have no idea what to order, I will skim the menu. As I am skimming the menu, the food that resonates most with me, will catch my attention like it is almost jumping off the page at me. This, to me, means that that particular food at that particular time is resonating with me so I order it. You may experience this *resonation* as a different sensation. Essentially, it makes itself known by standing out from all the rest of the other choices.

Narrowing the List

I now would like you to apply this experience of *something resonating* to your self-care list. To start this next step in the simple self-care journey, take a look at your list. Somewhere on this list is your one simple self-care that resonates the most with you. Ready to find it?

You have your self-care list in front of you. [See PAGE 48] Depending on the number of self-care you have written down, you may find it a little overwhelming. If you are feeling somewhat overwhelmed, this is natural. Rest assured that we will work through this together to simplify and find your one new thing.

First - Process of Elimination: Scan over your list and cross out the self-care that would take more time then you have available right now and the self-care that really does not appeal to you at this moment. Maybe the cost of a particular self-care isn't in your budget right now. Following, is an example of what your list may look like after the elimination step. By using the table of self-care from the previous section, I arbitrarily omitted things seen in gray and have added some of the simple self-care from the last section in **bold**. You get the idea. Work through your list and cross off whatever feels *not right* for this moment.

~~a nap~~	one glass of wine	being outside
~~aromatherapy~~	work on good posture	coloring
~~attending Taekwondo Class~~	knitting/needlework	join small church group
~~deep Breathing~~	running	walking
~~drink a smoothie~~	drink lots of water	drink water with lemon
~~drumming~~	warm cup of tea	Epsom salt bath
~~floss daily~~	~~walk with a buddy~~	7-9 hours of sleep
hiking	~~walking your dog~~	listening to soothing music
lifting weights	~~biking~~	~~cycling class~~
mantras	~~nutritional eating~~	10 min quiet time
massage	~~chiropractic~~	yoga
~~pedicure~~	~~facials~~	~~manicure~~
~~Pilates~~	~~bubble bath~~	stretching
~~practice taekwondo~~	talk with a friend/ sister	~~10 squats daily~~
~~reading fiction~~	reading scripture	journaling
~~singing~~	meditating	chanting
sunshine	dancing	playing with the kids
supplements	motivational quotes	positive affirmations
tai chi	joining a book club	line dancing
attend church regularly	counseling	drink green juice
Ragdoll pose	**being mindful**	**few more steps**
Stretch/brushing teeth	**ice wraps**	**gratitude journal**
foam roller	**reach up and out**	**deep breaths**

Please note: I am not implying that any of the self-care that is crossed out is less important than the ones not crossed out. All self-care is an important part of your life, but for this moment your focus is to cross out the self-care that you may find overwhelming, not interesting, or just doesn't fit into your time schedule right now. The more you can focus in on what really resonates and appeals to you now, the easier it will be to find your one new thing.

Again, this is merely a guide and an example of what your list may look like. I cannot emphasize enough how much this process is about *you* and your list will probably look very, very different and it's perfectly OK!

Second – Highlight Your *Resonators*: After you have crossed out the self-care that does not work or interest you right now, read over your list again list and this time put a check mark, symbol, or highlight the simple self-care that really resonates with you. **Pick 5 to 10 things that appeal most to you right now.**

Again, what *to resonate* may look like for you ... one of simple self-care things you have on your list might *pop* out at you or seem to stand out more than some of the others. As you are reading through your list, there may be a few things that *feel* more right to you. Mark those ones. Maybe the thought of "I would like to do that right now" may pop into your head. Be aware of the subtle signs your brain and body may be sending you. I hope this makes sense! This process may look and feel very different from one person to the next.

Below is an example of your list after highlighting your resonators.
Pick your top 5 – 10 choices.

a nap	one glass of wine	being outside
aromatherapy	work on good posture	coloring
attending Taekwondo Class	knitting/needlework	join small church group
deep Breathing	running	walking
drink a smoothie	***drink lots of water**	drink water with lemon
drumming	warm cup of tea	Epsom salt bath
floss daily	walk with a buddy	***7-9 hours of sleep**
hiking	walking your dog	listening to soothing music
*lifting weights	biking	cycling class
mantras	nutritional eating	10 min quiet time
massage	chiropractic	yoga
pedicure	facials	manicure
Pilates	bubble bath	stretching
practice taekwondo	talk with a friend/ sister	10 squats daily
reading fiction	reading scripture	journaling
singing	meditating	chanting
sunshine	dancing	playing with the kids
supplements	motivational quotes	positive affirmations
tai chi	joining a book club	line dancing
attend church regularly	counseling	drink green juice
*ragdoll pose	***being mindful**	***few more steps**
*stretch brushing teeth	***ice wraps**	***gratitude journal**
foam roller	***reach up and out**	deep breaths

Write these highlighted self-care choices below in the space provided. These 5 to 10 choices will now become your *new* list to work from:

_____

_____

_____

_____

_____

_____

_____

_____

_____

_____

> # *When you are stuck in a spiral,*
> # *to change all aspects of the spin,*
> # *you need only change one thing.*
>
> ## *~ Christina Baldwin*

Step 3: Just One Thing

Diverting here for a moment ... this always strikes me as funny and happens quite often during a workshop or seminar, AND I also fall victim to this way of thinking myself. At the end of the session, I typically ask each participant to pick *one* self-care to focus on for the next week, month, or until our next meeting. Inevitably, at least one woman will give me her *two* or *three* choices! Really, I said one! Picking only *one* is the most important basic principle that makes the simple self-care process work. One. Ladies, I said just one!

Like I said, I catch myself doing this quite often as well when I am needing to refocus on my self-care. Why can we not just pick one? Why do we feel we need to take on so much more than we are asked? Imagine the freedom if we just had one thing to focus on. Not two or three or four things, but one simple thing. I suppose I have made my point about picking just and only **one** thing! If after a few days, few weeks, or months of consistently doing your one new thing, then by all means, pick another!

By choosing just one thing, you are keeping things simple and doable. The whole point is to *not* to create overwhelm in your life, but to make your life a little more simple. Let's set ourselves up for *success* instead of setting ourselves up for failure.

Remember the definition of insanity ... *doing the same things over, and over again expecting different results.* So, when we make just one small change in our usual routine, it causes a shift in our habits allowing for different outcomes.

For example, several years ago I started stretching my hip flexors while brushing my teeth. This stretch, over time, has resulted in a decrease in my lower back discomfort during the rest of the day. I continue to do this stretch daily and often several times a day. Because I am in less pain, my mood has improved, and I have become a little less irritable and moody. Because I am in a better mood, my relationships at home go a little smoother and I have an overall better day. Because I am now happier and feel like I have a little more control over my back pain, I now feel like going for a walk in the morning which further improves my mood and well-being and so on. Because of the decreased discomfort, I feel a little more sense of control over my pain and this gives me a small boost of self-confidence.

If we take on too big of a change or too many things at one time:

   a. we're going to quit within a short amount of time because it's too much to keep up with,

   b. we will get tired really, fast and quit, or

   c. we will never get started because it is too overwhelming.

Just *one* thing.

I think it's pretty simple to slide one thing into your day without adding any stress to your life. Focusing on only one thing is soooo much easier that having to worry about several things to do as our plates are pretty much full already.

Over time, this becomes the turning point and will lead to other choices, one at a time as not to overwhelm. Remember: this is a journey ... a process, not a race. This is your journey and it may take 1 month to where you want to be or maybe three months or three years, but you know what?! In three frigging years, you are gonna be there, my friend. How powerful is that?!

Now, look at refined list of 5 to 10 choices. Read it over once or even twice. Just stare at it, if that works for you. Which one thing jumps out at you over all others? This, my friend, is the one thing you will start sliding into your day. This is your simple self-care to start your journey.

Write it Down: _____

MAKING IT WORK WITH MENTAL ROADBLOCKS

Oops ... a setback?! No worry!
NOW is a new moment to get
up and keep on trying again and
again and again!

Permission

As with any transformational personal journey, we will run into obstacles. No one said life would be easy and unfortunately, positive change does take some work. In this section, I am offering some solutions to, what I believe, are common roadblocks. Yes, we can run into them, turn around and go back the way we came or we can figure out how to get through them. I hope you find this section helpful.

Oddly enough, I think we sometimes need to give ourselves permission to take care of us. Yes, I know we are grown women. Yes, I know we make hundreds (maybe thousands) of decisions every day that impact, not only ourselves, but our children, spouses, partners, businesses, and our very existence, but yet why, oh why, do we feel like we don't *deserve* to take care of ourselves? Why do we feel like we are not *worthy* of some self-love in the form of self-care? If you know the answer, I would love to hear it! I'm still trying to figure that one out.

Believe it or not, this is a common feeling among women. I hear it quite often from women attending my workshops and MeetUp groups. Common comments include: "I feel like I don't deserve to do things for myself", or "I feel guilty if I take time for myself", or "I always put others before me." Where these feelings evolved from or how, I have no idea, but they seem to be quite ingrained in our female population.

Here is a simple suggestion to remind you that you are, in fact, allowed to take care of *you*! Here is a permission slip. Yes, a permission slip. And you thought only kids needed them! Simply fill in the blanks, read aloud, and sign. If you have an accountability buddy or good friend, have her be your witness and have her sign it as well. Let me ask you something … if you don't take care of you, who will?

My Permission Slip:

I, _____, *give myself permission to take time*
         (*fill in your name*)

for me and my self-care. In order to take care of others, I must take care of me first. I am worthy and I deserve my care and love as much as anyone else does. I give myself permission to show kindness and compassionate to myself. I promise to be understanding and patient with myself as I love and approve of myself.

Signed: _____

Witness: _____

Program Founder: Rita K. Garnto

Date: _____

Now photocopy and tape it to a place you will see it often and serve as a reminder. Your bathroom mirror or fridge can be great places. Want something a little less *public*? How about in your closet right beside your favorite clothes or shoes, home office, or another place that only you typically frequent?

Suggested Use: When you start to notice the same feelings of "I don't deserve time for myself", or "I feel guilty for taking time for me," re-surfacing in your mental chatter, re-read this permission slip out loud again and again. Remind yourself that you are *allowed* and do *deserve* to take care of you! If you don't, no one else will!

Success ... here I come!

The Why

I find if I have a definite purpose or motivation behind my decision and my choice, then I am more likely to keep with it and persevere. For some women, the driving force behind perseverance is having a strong *why*. *Why* are you wanting to make a change in your life? *Why* are you reading this book? *Why* are you not feeling good about yourself? It can also be a *what*. *What* gets you out of bed in the morning? *What* makes you want to make a change in your life? *What* is bothering you about your life?

Another name for your why or what is your *a-ha moment*. This is the moment you realize you really want or need to make a change. It clicks. The lightbulb goes off. The epiphany. I believe these a-ha moments can give you the drive and determination to start something new and, more importantly, keep going.

Some background thinking: By digging deeper into the real reason behind the desire for making a change can fuel the motivation to stick with your change long enough to turn a good new habit into a positive regular habit. I guarantee you that you will falter and stumble at some point with this new one thing and that is so ok because you are human after all!!

By defining and really understanding *why* you want to take better care of yourself, will help motivate you when you are stressed, overwhelmed, or maybe just tired. At these times, it is so very easy to fall back into your old ways of acting and thinking and sabotaging yourself. Just crown me the *Queen of Self-Sabotage*. By having a strong reason to stick to your change, can mean the difference between success and failure.

For example, one of my favorite go-to stress foods is dark chocolate. One or two pieces eaten mindfully can be a good stress reliever and good for you, but consuming a whole bar, not so much! When stressed I will grab a piece or two or four or even more. Before I know it, the whole bar is gone. Yikes! This habit is not helping me towards my goal of dropping a few pounds and this behavior is adding to my sense of lack of control, guilt, and shame.

Here's a different outcome of the same scenario by having a strong *why* in place. Same stressful situation and I go to get some dark chocolate. I pause and remind myself of my why I want to lose a few pounds ... with every extra pound of weight I carry, that is 4 extra pounds of pressure on my arthritic knees with every step. Do I still want some chocolate? Yes. I break off a piece or two. Put the rest back in the cupboard. Sit down and take time to enjoy it. Yum! I want more. I remind myself of those 4 extra pounds of pressure on my poor little knees and decide to walk back and forth to the mailbox or take three deep breaths instead or even drink a glass of water. Same scenario. Different outcome with less guilt and more sense of control. This is just one example of something I deal with. Yours can look very different and I hope you get the idea.

Take a moment to discover what your *go-to* thing is. Is it potato chips, ice-cream, wine, shopping? Awareness is such a powerful tool for making positive change.

My Favorite *Go-To*: _____

Let's get back to finding your *a-ha moment*. Your *why* can also be reframed into your *what*. What is going to:

a. keep you on track,

b. help get you back on track when you stumble.

For this next section, grab a writing utensil and journal, notebook, piece of paper, or just write on these pages. Read these questions over and answer the ones that resonate with you or seem more meaningful to you. There is no right or wrong. This is your process to finding the motivator(s) that will help you persevere and succeed. Again, not all the questions need to be answered. Look at the ones that resonate the most with you.

Questions to ask yourself:

Why am I starting this simple self-care journey? Because:

- I am tired of being tired
- To feel better
- To have more energy
- To lose weight
- To get into better shape
- Tone my muscles/legs/abs
- My blood pressure is high and I don't want to go on medication
- Run a marathon/half-marathon/5K
- I have a strong family history of heart disease/cancer/mental health issues/diabetes _____
- I want to see my children grow up/graduate/get married/meet my grandchildren
- I feel horrible about myself and want to make a change
- I want to be able to keep up with my kids

_____

_____

_____

_____

_____

WHAT is going to keep me moving forward with my one new thing:

_____

_____

_____

_____

_____

_____

HOW am I motivated:

_____

_____

_____

_____

_____

_____

_____

The RESULTS I want from this simple self-care change:

- Feel empowered
- Have more control over my life circumstances
- Take better care of myself
- Allow more time for ME
- Better health
- Better mood
- Become a nicer person
- More energy
- Healthier personal boundaries
- Better relationships

- Complete a triathlon

_____

_____

_____

_____

_____

Write down your *a-ha moment, why, or what* statement. What is your reason for wanting to make a positive change in your life?

_____

_____

_____

_____

_____

> *I am not perfect nor will I ever be.*
> *I am a work in progress, and that is*
> *definitely good enough!*

Not Good Enough and FALSE Expectations

Why is it that we can objectively look at our BFF, see her faults, as well as her strengths, and tell her how wonderful she is with honesty and love and **yet**, we do not treat ourselves with the same respect and love? She has faults and issues just like you do and yet you can create a space of acceptance and love for her. Why do we treat ourselves so differently? We are wonderful too, even with our faults and issues AND we deserve our own self-acceptance and self-love. Don't you think?!

Before we go any further I would like to clear up some of the *clutter of negativity* that may be living in your head. I like to refer to this less-than-positive clutter in my head as *my gremlins*. These gremlins are simply *my fears and insecurities* I have characterized, named, and given them a face. Three of my favorites are *Aunt Xiety*, *Notgooda Nuff*, and *Dissa Pointed* complete with portraits done by yours truly. (If you would like to learn more about gremlins, there is a great book by Rick Carson about taming your gremlins – see the resource section for info).

Sometimes, I just call these gremlins my *inner bitch*. You may very well have another name for these negative ninnies that feed on your fears and insecurities, but it's all pretty much the same useless, counter-productive, and worthless information taking up space inside your beautiful brain. When I get bogged down by the weight of my negativity, I affectionately refer to this gloomy mental state as *being stuck under my poop pile*. Grab your shovels, ladies! It is time to clear some of this shit out.

These gremlins, negative ninnies, inner bitches, fears, insecurities … however you want to name them, can manifest into an assortment of false expectations we place on ourselves. These false expectations then can evolve into a sense of being *not good enough*. Which is rather ironic because our fears and insecurities are actually there to protect us from getting hurt and making mistakes. But somehow their messages of protection have turned into messages of self-depreciation.

"I'm not good enough to be successful." "I'm not good enough to love." "I'm not good enough to try to lose weight." "I don't deserve to take care of myself."

I'm not good enough to _____
_____ .

(fill in the blank)

Unfortunately, our lists can go on and on. Eventually, this wears down our self-esteem, self-confidence, and self-worth. We truly can be our own worst enemy. Then, to add insult to injury we have the constant bombardment of society's messages laced with unrealistic ideals and images. It's not our fault that we often live under this false sense of not being good enough. As part of my research for this book, I posted this question on Facebook:

If you were to create a list of negative comments that creep into your head when you are not feeling great about yourself, what would they look like?

Here are some of the responses directly quoted from the many women that replied:

- I'm a terrible leader
- They don't listen to me
- I'm so fat
- What's wrong with me
- I'm just not doing it right
- Coulda, Shoulda, Woulda----

- How would life be different if I attended a four-year college or had a degree?
- I'm a failure
- I didn't do enough
- I never complete anything
- I'm so mean
- I hate my voice
- I'm such a push over
- I'm too selfish. I should do more for others.
- For not being able to put a good dinner together.
- I should get more done
- I should be skinny to be noticed to be seen to be successful
- If I am not skinny I am not beautiful
- To be loved enough I have to be better, thinner, successful
- I wish I could get more organized in my physical space and 'head' space. I'm a list maker but often get overwhelmed with the 'to do list', I find myself saying to self, 'screw it' – I'll do it tomorrow, weekend, next week.
- And of course, wish I were fit – fell off the workout wagon when I hurt my back. Thinner would be nice, but for me, regular work-outs help!
- I'm too different...people won't like my creative take on my designs. I'm just not good enough to succeed in this business!
- I waste time. I don't exercise enough. I'm lazy
- I have big thighs, big butt, bubble butt

If these replies do not scream an "I'm not good enough" attitude then I don't know what does. I think this is also proof that we are not alone in how we feel and it shows that we have a much bigger social issue that is running rampant.

Another goal I have is to create a sense of support and community among us like-minded women. I think for too long we have been pitted against one another thinking that if I make you out to be less than me than I will automatically be better. Nope! Doesn't work that way. Building one another up and supporting one another, I think, really is the answer to creating a more loving and supportive environment for all of us.

Back to ... not being good enough. Are you still not sure what I am talking about? Take a look at the following question and answer it honestly:

When you see your friends on Facebook and all their awesome posts. What is your first reaction?

A. well, my life sucks!

B. Why can't I be as fabulous as her?

C. What am I doing wrong?

D. What is wrong with me?

E. Why am I such a failure?

F. All of the above

If you picked *any* of the answers, then, my dear, there is some negativity clutter filling your head space and maybe even a gremlin or two. Let's break down this negativity clutter into what I will call our *FALSE* belief system. In this case, FALSE refers to:

*F*ear *A*ttracts *L*ots of **S*enseless *E*xpectations.

(*Feel free to insert any "S" word ... silly, stupid, shitty ... you get the idea.)

It really says it all. Our beliefs about ourselves are often false statements that we have decided to adopt as our truths based on non-truths and perceptions of past events from childhood and adulthood.

Now, let's take a look at your FALSE list. Just like your story, your FALSE (Fear Attracts Lots of Senseless Expectations) belief system will be unique and different because it is made up of your experiences, memories, moments, and your life.

In case you are still not sure what your FALSE belief system looks like, read on and fill in the blanks below. Be honest with your answer(s) please. Pick as many as applicable.

"Because I cannot effectively _____,

Fill in the blank with any of the following choices:

jump out of bed energetically in the morning, control my food cravings, clean my house regularly, run my business, take care of my kids, keep my Quickbooks up to date, drive my kids to all their extracurricular activities, be a sex kitten every night for my partner, cook, do laundry, buy groceries, exercise regularly, keep my youthful figure, and oh ya, get enough sleep.

I am *not a good enough* _____!"

Fill in the above blank with any of the following choices:

Mom, wife, business owner, employee, cook, sex kitten, friend, person, human being, 40-60 year old trying to maintain my 25 year old body that I had before having kids and/or entering menopause, or any other noun you find appropriate.

Yes, this is a little tongue in cheek and sounds a little silly. I hope you can see how sometimes we have these kinda crazy, unrealistic expectations that just cannot be lived up to. Why? Because that is not real life. Life is hard and then, can get even harder. Rest assured that none of us ... and I repeat none of us will ever have a chance in hell of ever living up to the false expectations that we create in our heads. It's time to do what they sang about in the movie Frozen. *LET IT GO!*

Pause. Take a deep breath. In ... count ... 1, 2, 3 ... hold 1, 2, 3 ... out 1, 2, 3

Repeat after me. *I am good enough!* If this phrase resonates with you, write it on a sticky note and put it on your bathroom mirror as a reminder.

I suggest that you take a few minutes to examine your FALSE belief system and maybe even write them down on a piece of paper or in your journal. Ready to start getting rid of them? Take the piece of paper and rip it, burn it, shred it, or flush it down the toilet. Literally get rid of your list.

I think awareness is the key to making positive changes in our lives. If we become aware of our thought patterns, behaviors, habits, then we can consciously change them.

Giving up on your goal because of one setback is like slashing your other three tires because you got one flat.

It Doesn't Have to be All or Nothing

I grew up with an *all or nothing personality,* as in, I was either dieting, depriving myself, working out like crazy, or eating whatever I wanted and not working out. In my early 20's, I could do that and do it well. (Interestingly enough, in my twenties, I based my day, whether it was a good day or a bad day, strictly on my food choices and whether the food choices were *good* or *bad*.) Very sad especially when I think about all the energy I wasted on such an abstract thought pattern. It is amazing the dysfunctional thought patterns we can acquire as we get older.

You might be wondering how do I remember that far back. Well, really it was only 30ish years ago. Ya, my memory is not *that* good. I still have my journals from back then to prove it. When I started rereading those journals from 20, 30 years ago, I was so saddened by the amount of energy I wasted on thinking I was fat, not good enough, or if "I just lost 10 pounds" life would be so much better. I am saddened by the amount of living I missed out on because I was so focused on these negative messages instead of loving me for who I was.

Even though I feel like I wasted so much time in my past with some poor choices, I have no regrets for any of those choices. Why? Because if I hadn't gone through all that stuff and worked through those negative thoughts and lived my life I the way I did, I would not be sitting here writing this book. Our stories make us who we are today and will shape who we become tomorrow.

Over time I have come to realize that moderation is so much better and more effective over the long run. Yes, with all or nothing, you could have very quick results – both positive and negative, but it didn't allow for enjoying life. Let me explain. When I was in the *all mode*, I solely focused on dieting and working out. My whole schedule focused on those two things and I didn't go out with friends and socialize because it was *all* about getting into shape. When I was in the *nothing mode*, I ate everything that I could think of and did not work out at all. All this eating didn't make me feel good mentally or physically and the lack of any real exercise contributed to feeling icky. Yes, I packed on the pounds too and all my hard work from my *all* phase was quickly eradicated.

If I had opted a more moderate approach, I could have eaten in moderation still enjoying some of the *treat* foods, worked out regularly instead of fanatically, and socialized without guilt. I'm guessing I would have been much happier and more satisfied with my life at the time.

The theory of *consistent moderation* as opposed to *all or nothing* will pay off in the long run. I am reminded of how well consistency and moderation work whenever I think of my friend that lost over 160 pounds in three years. It wasn't fast and I know it wasn't easy, but she was consistent and she did it! That is the beauty and power of consistency, moderation, positive thinking, and intention. It works over time and the only person you have to convince of that, is *you!*

SECTION 5

MAKING IT WORK WITH TOOLS

For right now let's talk about different tools you may find helpful to not only get started, but to start on track on your simple self-care journey. Again, it's all about what resonates with you. My hope to is give you more tools in your tool belt so when the going gets tough and you start wavering, you'll have something to remind you why you started in the first place and why it is so important to keep going.

Journaling is like whispering to one's self and listening at the same time.

~ Mina Murray, Dracula

Journaling

There is a certain strength and power in putting your thoughts down on paper. There is something so cleansing about getting *that stuff* out of your head. Often when I journal, I feel like I have had a conversation with a good friend. Now, that may sound a little weird to you as this conversation is clearly one-sided, but I am constantly amazed at the clarity I gain from getting my thoughts out of my head onto paper. Solutions to current issues may all of a sudden appear in front of me or the turmoil in my head calms down with the ultimate result being that I can think clearer, I am less stressed, and I can function better.

If journaling is one those things that resonates with you, here are some guidelines to getting you started. To be completely honest with you, I do not journal every day. I would love to on some level, but that doesn't always work out. However, I know that when I am feeling down, frustrated, even excited, or just having a poopy day, by journaling I can turn my day around.

The Steps to Journaling:

1. **Choosing a Journal**

   Your journal can be a blank book, notebook, designer journal with lines or unlined. An app on your laptop can also serve as your journal.

2. **Set Aside Time**

   This is probably one of the most difficult aspects unless you create a habit of writing at the same time. It really is all about finding a time that works for *you* whether it is morning, evening, lunch break, or bedtime, it has to work for *you.* I like to call this finding *your pocket of time* to write.

3. **Begin Writing**

   Don't think about what to write, or how to write or if it sounds stupid or not ... just write! You are the only one going to be reading this. Grammar, punctuation, spelling . . . no worries! It doesn't matter.

4. **What to Write**

   Suggestions include writing about your feelings and thoughts surrounding emotional events, venting negative emotions, cataloging events, making lists, and even reliving events emotionally. Try to let solutions to situations you're facing *flow* from your pen as you write.

5. **Keep Your Journal Private**

   When talking with other women, the security of the journal is a common concern. Finding a secure *hiding place* for your journal, changing hiding spots regularly, and not sharing with others that you are keeping a journal are the most obvious options. Other options include buying a journal with a lock or storing it in a lock box or safe of some sort. If you are using your laptop, using a secure password to safely guard its privacy is an easy solution. If you are really concerned about someone finding your writings especially after an extremely emotional event, simply burn, shred, or tear up the paper you have written on after you are done writing. It is amazing how cleansing and therapeutic destroying what you have written can be.

6. Other Simple Tips

- Get in the habit of writing in your journal
- Don't worry about neatness - just get your thoughts and feelings down on paper
- Do *not* self-censor; let go of any *shoulds, coulds, or woulds*. Just write what you feel like writing.
- Like Nike says ... ***just do it!!***

Gratitude Journal - Living in Gratitude

Keeping a gratitude journal is taking journaling and simplifying it a little more. The first I heard about this was from Oprah when she still had her regular talk show. If you are stuck with not knowing what to write or how to start writing in your journal, try this simple practice. Write 3 to 5 things that you are grateful for. This could be as simple as having food to eat, a roof over your head, a job, a supportive partner, or a bed to sleep in. Maybe you have had a great opportunity come up today or met a person that may lead to some great sales. Did someone pay you an unexpected compliment? Did you manage not to step in all that goose poop on the sidewalk as you went for your morning stroll? Remember to set up the coffee on auto pilot so it was ready when you got up? Keep it simple sweetie! Just be grateful.

What I really like about this kind of journaling is the positive awareness and mindful piece it can bring to your thought patterns. It takes just a moment. There is something about the pausing, looking around, and really noticing all the positive things you have in your life that can nudge you out of any funk you might be in. When I go for my morning walk with my dogs, I try really hard to walk in a mindset of gratitude. I notice the sky and am grateful it's not raining or look at all the blooming trees and flowers. Take a deep breath and look around. Give it a try! You may be very surprised with the result.

Mind Over Matter - if you don't mind, it doesn't matter.

Mental Motivation

Over the years, I have used different methods of mental motivation. I have found 3 types of mental motivation that have worked for me at various times in the past. I may use all them in a day or maybe just one. They are creative visualizations, mantras, and inspirational quotes.

Creative Visualization

Creative Visualizations, according to well-known author of creative visualization books, Shakti Gawain, are defined as *the practice of seeking to affect the outer world by changing one's thoughts and expectations.*

Shakti Gawain writes in her book, *Creative Visualization,* one of the ways to use creative visualization is to first choose something you wish to attain or achieve. Now using your imagination, see yourself having it and experience the feelings, the gratitude, sharing it with friends, and admiring it. This is really a very powerful technique and the following is an excerpt from her book.

Creative Visualization: A Simple Exercise in Creative Visualization
Shakti Gawain ©

Here is an exercise in the basic technique of creative Visualization:

First, think of something you would like. For this exercise choose something simple, that you can easily imagine attaining. It might be an object you would like to have, an event you would like to have happen, a situation in which you'd like to find yourself, or some circumstance in your life you'd like to improve.

Get in a comfortable position, either sitting or lying down, in a quiet place where you won't be disturbed. Relax your body completely. Starting from your toes and moving up to your scalp, think of relaxing each muscle in your body in turn, letting all tension flow out of your body. Breathe deeply and slowly, from your belly. Count down slowly from ten to one, feeling yourself getting more deeply relaxed with each count.

When you feel deeply relaxed, start to imagine the thing you want exactly as you would like it. If it is an object, imagine yourself with the object, using it, admiring it, enjoying it, showing it to friends. If it is a situation or event, imagine yourself there and everything happening just as you want it to. You may imagine what people are saying, or any details that make it more real to you.

You may take a relatively short time or quite a few minutes to imagine this-whatever feels best to you. Have fun with it. It should be a thoroughly enjoyable experience, like a child daydreaming about what he wants for his birthday.

Now, keeping the idea or image still in your mind, mentally make some very positive, affirmative statements to yourself (aloud or silently, as you prefer) about it, such as:

Here I am spending a wonderful weekend in the mountains. What a beautiful vacation. Or I love the view from my spacious, new apartment. Or I'm learning to love and accept myself as I am.

These positive statements, called affirmations, are a very important part of creative visualization, which I discuss in more detail later.

If you like, you can end your visualization with the firm statement to yourself:

This, or something better, now manifests for me in totally satisfying and harmonious ways, for the highest good of all concerned.

This statement leaves room for something different and even better than you had originally envisioned happening, and serves as a reminder to you that this process only functions for the mutual benefit of all.

If doubts or contradictory thoughts arise, don't resist them or try to prevent them. This will tend to give them a power they don't otherwise have. Just let them flow through your consciousness, acknowledge them, and return to your positive statements and images.

Do this process only as long as you find it enjoyable and interesting. It could be five minutes or half an hour. Repeat every day, or as often as you can.

As you see, the basic process is relatively simple. Using it really effectively, however, usually requires some understanding and refinement.

(From the book *Creative Visualization*. Copyright © 2002, 1995, 1978 by Shakti Gawain. Reprinted with permission of New World Library, Novato, CA. www.newworldlibrary.com)

Take a moment to jot down some topics for creative visualizations that you would find helpful. Examples can include anything from visualizing yourself getting up early to work out or meditate to staying calm in a stressful situation to feeling confident while delivering a power keynote speech to confronting a difficult person in a positive way. The sky is the limit! Maybe there is a bad habit you would like to change. What would that look like? Write down some of your stumbling blocks you want to overcome.

_____

_____

_____

_____

Mantras

Mantras are defined as *an often repeated word, formula, or phrase.* Your mantra may not necessarily be true at the moment, but rather, something you are wishing to manifest and make happen. Your mantra can be used to stop and change the destructive messaging your negative self-talk and thoughts are perpetuating. I find this method very good at silencing my gremlins and fears. They can also be used to motivate and overcome difficult moments, doubts, and fear. Examples I frequently use are: *Yes, I can with ease*, and *I love and approve of myself.*

A true story to show you the power of positive mantras. I had moved to NC from Saudi Arabia and I was looking for a new job. I was looking at relocating to the Charlotte area and I applied for the job of *Transport Respiratory Therapist*. Apparently, I did not read all the fine print as I was very unprepared for the job interview. I assumed, quite incorrectly, that the interview would last about an hour or so and the interview was for the job of transporting patients in the back of an ambulance from hospital to hospital. The only thing I got right was the transporting part.

I show up to the interview along with several others and come to find out that the interview would be FOUR hours long and it would start with a quiz. Not just any quiz, mind you, it was quiz consisting of ten EKG (heart rhythm) strips that we were required not only to identify and name correctly, but also breakdown the rhythms into their components with the time increments. Since that wasn't enough stress, we were told there would then be FOUR oral testing stations where two members of the flight team would grill each of us on very specific emergency situations. OMG! Really?!

Needless to say, I was very overwhelmed and basically, freaking out. I went to the bathroom and sat in a stall and I went through my options. One, I could walk out the front of the hospital never to be seen again or two, I could stay and do my best. To be very honest with you, the front door option was looking really good, but was very against the grain of my character. I then began a repeating a mantra that I had been given years before by my massage therapist in Vancouver.

I love and approve of myself.
I am safe where I am.
I create my own security.
I am at peace with my own feelings.

I repeated this over and over and over again while I was seated in the potty. Quite the visual! After my nerves had calmed down a little, I left the stall (washed my hands, of course) and proceeded to the interview.

At this point, all I could do was my best. Much to my surprise, I was hired along with several others and spent the next three and half years in a very exciting, fulfilling, and emotionally charged job. To this day, I feel truly blessed that I was given the opportunity to be part of such an amazing group of people.

Do you have any favorite mantras? If you are stuck, google *mantras to live by* and you be surprised what you find that resonates with you. Louise Hay, well-known motivational author, has written a multitude of books including *You Can Heal Your Life*. This book is full of wonderful mantras. Write your mantra down below.

Suggested Use: Copy on a sticky note and stick it to your mirror or fridge or copy on an index card and carry it with you.

My Mantra is: _____
_____
_____
_____
_____
_____
_____

Inspirational Quotes

Inspirational quotes are the third type of mental motivation I want to mention. Inspirational quotes can be a very powerful tool with motivation. The ripple effect a good quote can have, never ceases to amaze me. There are two quotes that immediately come to mind that helped shape my passion for self-care education.

One is written by Christina Baldwin – "When you are stuck in a spiral, to change all aspects of the spin, change just one thing." I have it taped to my mirror and it has been there for years. For some reason that quote so resonated for me and looking back I see that it was the catalyst that started my journey to developing my *just one thing* philosophy. It has, in fact, made such an impact on me that I have created my own quote based on her quote, *When you are mired in your muck, to start moving forward do just one new thing, one little thing.* Another one of my favorite quotes is from Kobi Yamada … *Be good to yourself. If you don't take care of your body, where will you live?*

What are some of your favorite quotes? Do you have them written down somewhere or posted on a wall or mirror? Having a favorite quote on your wall, or mirror can add a little inspiration to your day every time you see it. Sticky notes work really well and allow you to stick your quote where it best works for you … fridge, bathroom mirror, computer, car dashboard. I use dry erase maker to write on my bathroom mirror. (I used to use lipstick, but to be very honest, that made for one heck of clean up job when I wanted to change my message.)

Maybe you would like to start a *quote* journal. A journal or notebook strictly dedicated to favorite quotes. I started a quote journal when I moved to Saudi Arabia many years ago and still occasionally add quotes to it and go back and read over the quotes that have inspired me in the past.

I love quotes so much, in fact, that I have created a quote jar with the signature label, **I.C. Quotes**. (The I and C are the initials of my daughters and create a fun play on words.) Quote jars are a great way to get a random or maybe not-so-random message from the Universe. Pick a quote from the jar first thing in the morning or any time during the day when you need a little inspiration.

Want to make your own jar? It's easy to make your own. Simply print out your quotes, cut them into strips to separate them, fold into small shapes, and place them in your container. Any small container will do as long as the opening is large enough for your hand to reach inside. If you don't have the time or don't want to go through the trouble of making your own, you can order one of the *I.C. Quotes* Jars. Please see the resource section at the end of the book for ordering information.

> # *It is not only what we do, but also what we do not do, for which we are accountable.*
>
> ## *~ Moliere*

Accountability

Accountability systems can help you stay on target and keep on track. An accountability system can be as simple as keeping track of your activities and progress in a notebook, on a calendar, tracking sheet, or on your phone. Keeping a visual record of your accomplishments and progress can be a really great tool to help keep you motivated and actively engaged. This does not work for everyone. Again, this must resonate with you in order to be effective.

Using a calendar (one that has large blocks of white space around each date) is an inexpensive way to track your self-care can easily be printed off the computer. I started using the calendar system back in the early 1980's when I started working out at the gym. I simply wrote down what type of workout I did (cardio, weights, abdominals, stretches, etc.) on the appropriate day along with the minutes of cardio. I created a system of abbreviations that would allow a quick way to make note of everything. For example, I use *elip* for elliptical, *abs* for abdominal exercise, *S* for my stretching routine ... you get the idea. I encourage you to create your own system to simplify. If I didn't work out or do some self-care, I would draw a line diagonally through the day and leave it blank. I did *not* like to see lots of blank spaces with lines drawn through them on my calendar so that helped motivate me and get my hiney in gear to so something!

I now print out blank calendar months from my computer and tape them inside my side cabinet in the bathroom. I still do *not* like to see too many blank space with lines drawn through them! Still working for me! Would this work for you?

Examples of calendar pages and checklist can be found in the Resources section.

Do you fare better with human support? How about finding a buddy or accountability partner? With an accountability partner, you can check-in regularly with her and her with you. If you plan on doing activities together, such as regular walks, having a buddy will help you stay motivated. If you aren't wanting to do the activity, she can help get you out the door and vice versa. Plan a goal together and communicate regularly to make sure each other is staying on track.

Also, lots of technology is available to make it even easier if you are a tech-lover. There are all kinds of devices that will keep track of your steps to more elaborate, involved tracking health devices. I think the trick really is to find what will work for you. There are all kinds of meal tracking programs and so on. Too many for me to even try to keep up with. Do some exploring of your own and see what resonates with you and your life style.

New apps for your phone are popping up all the time. There are lots of free apps and ones that are low cost. Take some time to check it out and see what will work best for you. I use a simple step tracking device and have intentionally not upgraded to one that does more information gathering. I might in the future, but for right now this is working for me. Keeping it simple sweetie.

Below, list the devices that you are using or would like to use to help you keep track of your progress.

_____

_____

_____

Life is the journey of steps and not a destination.

A Day in the Life

WARNING: Before you read this, repeat after me ...

"This has taken Rita YEARS to get here to this place of integrated simple self-care. My ONLY purpose is to read this following list and imagine my life, too, could be filled with simple self-care in the years to come. My ONLY focus right now is to start with only ONE simple self-care choice that resonates with me!"

Please take a look at the list as individual simple self-care choices as opposed to "OMG! She does all that?!"

To give you an idea of what one of my days might look with simple self-care and self-care sprinkled throughout, here is an example of one of my typical days:

- ✓ Knees to Chest and *give myself a hug* before I get out of bed
- ✓ Roll over on my side and *get out of bed the right way*
- ✓ As I am walking to the bathroom, *reach up* and do gentle *shoulder rolls* to start getting the kinks out
- ✓ Drink a big glass of water
- ✓ Repeat my *mantra* written on my mirror

✓ *Stretch while brushing my teeth*

✓ While coffee is brewing, heat up my *flaxseed neck wrap* and place in on my tight shoulders ... ahhhh

✓ Grab my cup of coffee and sit for a moment of *mindfulness and gratitude*

✓ If I didn't sleep well and I am feeling irritable, I grab my *journal* and start writing to get whatever is bothering me out of my head. I will feel a little better after a few minutes

✓ Busy day ahead ... my kids are up for school and encourage them to get ready for their day. *Pause and deep breath* when I am met with their resistance and whining

✓ And say a quick *prayer* asking for patience

✓ Eat a good healthy breakfast, take my supplements, and drink more water

✓ Off to the school bus with my youngest daughter and grab the dogs and go for a 15-minute walk after she gets on the bus while listening to my favorite music playlist

✓ Off to my massage office to see clients

✓ I park at the far end of the parking lot so I take *a few more steps*

✓ As I set up my massage table, I walk around my massage table a few extra times for *few more steps* as well as do some knee raises and other simple movements

✓ Or maybe do *ragdoll* while waiting for client

✓ Grab a handful of almonds between clients and *drink more water*

✓ When I get home, put feet up and take 15 minutes of *quiet time* eating a good plant based lunch

✓ Go do some work on the computer

✓ For bathroom breaks, I go downstairs for a *few more steps*

✓ Kids home from school. Sit down and have snack with them and engage with them.

✓ Take an evening taekwondo class with hubbie and the kids

✓ After class, put velcro *ice wraps* on my knees so I can ice and make dinner at the same time

✓ Nighttime ritual of winding down & TV off 30 minutes before bedtime

✓ Get ready for bedtime

✓ As water in shower warms up, let cold water run on my knees

✓ Use my homemade lavender sugar scrub in the shower to help relax me and moisturize my skin

✓ *Stretch while I brush my teeth*

✓ While trying to get to sleep do a *creative visualization* about wanting to get up early before everyone else

✓ Sleep and repeat

My day typically contains lots of different simple self-care and your day may already have more than you realize. My routine now has evolved over the years of being conscious of doing self-care and finding and creating ways to add self-care into my life. By no means, are you to expect yourself to create a schedule like mine. Start with *one new thing, one little thing* only.

The philosophy of one: do one new thing, change just one little thing.

Recap - The 3 steps

Now it is your turn to take all the information that has resonated with you and start your own simple self-care transformation. Remember to start with just *one* thing! Here is a recap of the three steps to finding your one thing.

Step 1: Keep It Simple Sweetie

This was the information gathering step where you started the process for finding your one thing, the one new thing to begin the positive transformation and change you would like to see in your life.

By keeping this list simple, the journey is less overwhelming and much easier to follow. The *simple* piece is put into action by just grabbing a writing utensil and blank piece of paper, laptop, or, better yet, a journal or notebook and jotting down all the self-care that appeals to you. This becomes a beginning point that should not take much time or brain power. Just start writing. By writing down all the self-care you are *willing* to do, *can* do, and are *able* to do creates your self-care wish list. This is now your personalized go-to resource list.

Let's revisit the definition of **self-care**. It is defined as *any intentional action you take to care for your mental, emotional, physical and spiritual health.* The next piece to this step was adding the word **simple** to self-care and to start looking at (and adding to your list) the simple self-care that *is easy, not rocket science or complicated, and can easily* **slide** *into your busy day-to-day schedule.* See page 49. Lots of examples are found in the section titled *Simple Self-Care.* By adding to your list, any of these simple self-care suggestions and others that you may come across on the internet, hear from a friend, or create yourself, completes Step 1.

Step 2: It Must Resonate

Because this whole process is about *you,* when you start narrowing down your list, in order to be successful, these choices must *resonate* with you. There has to be some kind of *draw,* some kind of pull, or positive emotional connection to your choices in order for this to work.

For example, I love walking while listening to one of my favorite playlists. The music for that walk might be upbeat, high energy or it might be slower, more soulful, or maybe even Christian music. I have come to cherish this me time where my brain can go on a happy little journey wherever it wants. I may solve a problem, create a new keynote speech, just occupy a space of pure gratitude and joy during my walk, or just calm down after a stressful situation. I look forward to this time and because this choice really resonates with me, I find that I can get myself out the door even when I am exhausted, stressed, or crabby because I know it will make me feel better!

Creating your short list in step 2 gets rid of the extraneous self-care options that do not or cannot slide into your life at this moment. Maybe it just doesn't appeal to you right now. I suggest picking 5 to 10 to give you some freedom of choice, but feel free to pick only 3 for your short list. Again, it is *all about you!* Have your short list? Step 2 is now complete.

Step 3: Just One Thing

Our goal during this whole process is to set ourselves up for success *not* failure. It is easy to become overwhelmed by taking on too many things at once. (Ya, don't know anything about that?!) Hence, the step of picking only *one* thing. Taking your short list, read over your simple self-care choices and pick one. Yes, just one, my friend, just one. This one simple self-care is now your focus and your goal is to slide it into your day, every day!

> # *When you are mired in your muck, to get unstuck do one new thing, just change one little thing.*
>
> *~ Rita K Garnto*

In Closing

Yes, these steps and this process may seem over simplified and quite frankly, that is the point! ☺ In this day and age, simple is good! So now you have your one thing! Yay! Now what?

Look over the *Making It Work with Tools* section and pick the one tool that will help you get started and stay on track. Run into a mental roadblock? Reread the *Making It Work When with Mental Roadblocks* for possible solutions. Use journaling as problem solving and a source of solutions. You may surprise yourself!

Getting started is the easy part. It's the staying on track on a consistent basis that can be the challenging part. It is only hard until this new simple self-care becomes a habit, a part of your life schedule. The hope is that you will get to this point where if you *don't* do your simple self-care, you will actually miss it and it will feel like you have forgotten to do something. That is when you know you have arrived at your next step.

Your next step will be to pick another *one* simple self-care to add to your daily routine. Using your list you have already created in Step 1 and 2, find your one new thing and add it to your day keeping track just like you did with your first *one new thing*. Continue to repeat this process as your self-care plan evolves. Be consistent. Be persistent. Love yourself.

For more in-depth step-by-step tracking, please refer to the tracking sheets in the Resource section.

In a year, you may be very amazed when you look back to see how much your life has changed. I think, one of the most important things to remember is that life is a journey and a process. It is made up thousands and thousands of pieces. Do your best! That is all that any of us can promise ourselves.

I hope that you have found this book helpful in finding your one new thing, one little thing to start your simple self-care journey. Thank you for being part of my journey! I would love to hear what your *one new thing* is. Feel free to email me at rita@simpleselfcare.net and looking forward to hearing from you!

Happy self-caring,

Rita ☺

SECTION 7

RESOURCES

Worksheets

Instructions for Simple Self-Care Progress Tracking Sheet
https://goo.gl/jTFP63

14 Day Tracking Sheet
https://goo.gl/VPhk4C

Month Tracking Sheet
https://goo.gl/GMT59F

Accountability Tools

www.pdfcalendar.com
Excel calendar template

Ice Massage Description

The easiest way to perform ice massage is to use ice that has been frozen in a small paper cup. It is not a bad idea to keep one or two ice cups in the freezer for those unexpected injuries.

When you are ready to start, tear a small layer of the paper cup off to expose the ice. Place towel under the affected area. Apply the ice to the skin with circular motions. Keep the ice moving over the injured area for the entire time to prevent any frost bite and keep an eye on the time so as not to overdo it. I have found that a total of 5 minutes is effective even though I have read articles that state the ice massage can be done for up to 10 minutes. If anything, please err on the side of caution and start off with a shorter time until you see how your skin reacts.

Typically, ice massage will take you through 4 stages during application:

1. **Cold** when ice first applied
2. After a minute or two, a **burning** or **prickling** sensation may set in
3. Followed by an **aching** sensation (which may sometimes hurt more than the pain)
4. Then finally, the most important stage, **numbness**.

Once the skin feels numb to the touch, stop the ice massage. Allow the iced body part to warm up naturally. Put the remaining ice in the freezer to save for the next application.

This process can be repeated several times during the day, making sure to always allow the area of ice application to completely **warm-up** between applications so as not to cause skin irritation and/or frostbite.

For more information, talk to your healthcare professional specifically your physical therapist and/or massage therapist.

Signature Self-Care Products

For more information regarding the signature self-care products and to order the organic neck wraps, IC Quotes Jar, and other great simple self-care products, I invite you to visit my website http://simpleselfcare.net.

Information Sources

Duhigg, Charles. The Power of Habit. New York: Random House, 2012

"self-care". *Dictionary.com Unabridged*. Random House, Inc. 23 Jan. 2017. Dictionary.com http://www.dictionary.com/browse/self-care.

Carson, Rick. Taming Your Gremlin (Revised Edition): A Surprisingly Simple Method for Getting Out of Your Own Way. New York: Harper Collins, 2009

Nelson, Arnold G. & Kokkonen Jouko. Stretching Anatomy. Champaign: Human Kinetics, 2007

Anderson, Bob. Stretching. Bolinas: Shelter Publications, 2010

Bery, Kristian. Prescriptive Stretching. Champaign: Human Kinetics, 2011

Cabane, Olivia Fox. The Charisma Myth. New York: Penguin, 2012

Elaine N. Marieb RN, Ph.D. Human Anatomy & Physiology, Fifth Edition. United States: Benjamin Cummings, an imprint of Addison Wesley Longman, Inc., 2001

https://www.stress.org/what-is-stress/

From the book *Creative Visualization*. Copyright © 2002, 1995, 1978 by Shakti Gawain. Reprinted with permission of New World Library, Novato, CA. www.newworldlibrary.com

http://www.livestrong.com/article/290889-what-size-stability-ball-should-i-buy/

Hay, Louise L., You Can Heal Your Life. Carson, CA: Hay House Inc., 1984

ABOUT THE AUTHOR

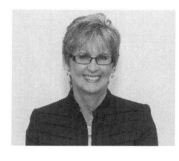

Rita K. Garnto lives in Charlotte, NC with her husband, two daughters, 2 dogs, and 2 cats. She is currently maintaining her private massage therapy practice with plans to retire from massage at the end of 2018. Her future plans include spending more quality time with family, writing more books, traveling, live seminars, speaking engagements, webinars, and continuing with her own simple self-care.

With a personal journey filled with many challenges including infertility, adoption, family death, and chronic health issues, Rita is no stranger to extreme stress. Based on her own health struggles plus 35+ years of healthcare experience, Rita, as the Simple Self-Care Mentor and Educator, has developed her own self-care philosophy and the steps to obtain a better quality of health using simple self-care.

Rita's mantra is "When you are mired in your muck, to get unstuck do one new thing, just one little thing." She wants women to understand how powerful just one small change can be and how large of an impact it can have on their future health and well-being. Rita shares her story and philosophy through a variety of presentations and interactive workshops as well as one-on-one mentoring. By sharing her story of perseverance and self-care, she hopes to inspire and show women how to put themselves on the top of their to-do lists with their simple self-care choices.

Made in the USA
San Bernardino, CA
26 March 2018